Instant Gratification

Mastering the Art of Overcoming Instant Gratification

(Reduce Instant Gratification, Beat Social Media Addiction, and Stop Wasting Your Life)

Anthony Bowen

Published By **Ryan Princeton**

Anthony Bowen

All Rights Reserved

Instant Gratification: Mastering the Art of Overcoming Instant Gratification (Reduce Instant Gratification, Beat Social Media Addiction, and Stop Wasting Your Life)

ISBN 978-1-9995502-8-8

Legal & Disclaimer

Table Of Contents

Chapter 1: What Exactly Is Pleasure?

What is the reason we feel it? What is the reason we feel pleasure and how do we cause it to happen? What is the reason we keep repeating the same patterns throughout our lives, after you have completed something different or that is repetitive, which makes us feel in a good and positive mood? It is the feeling that makes you feel good and that includes enjoying some thing. It is different from pain or suffering, which are the result of experiencing bad feelings. The pleasure itself - the good feeling that you feel when you eat or sex, as well as drugs is triggered by the release of various kinds of neurotransmitters (chemical messengers) throughout the brain. Dopamine production in the reward system of the brain is especially important. Dopamine releases informs that the brain to anticipate reward from something, and also controls the degree of reward and motivates us to look for satisfying objects. This is akin to pleasure. It's inextricably linked to desire, value and actions. Animals, including humans, feel pleasure is enjoyable, satisfying or worth looking for. The more rewarding a reward is, the more likely it is that you'll be able to repeat it again. There are a variety of things that can be described as enjoyable for example, eating, enjoying sexual relations while listening to music, engaging in games that allow you to get away from the reality. However, what's fascinating in pleasure is it is a challenge to describe what they enjoy. There is no one who can answer that pleasure only stems through instant rewards. It also includes a delay in time reward. Dopamine also plays a role in many other tasks including voluntary movements and cognitive. Schizophrenia-related disorders have an excessive release of dopamine, that can cause symptoms of psychosis. For neurodegenerative conditions like Parkinson's disease, dopamine-producing cells that are that are responsible for motor coordination stop dying quickly. Why would excessive dopamine increase cause? It doesn't, but it does rot each time we aren't sure what our boundaries are or how to enjoy the instant gratification, or delay satisfaction. In Chapter 6. "How we can improve" I've written about ways to get into the delayed gratification process in detail, and then how to maintain the positive habits. However, we'll discuss this later.

Well-being and happiness are tightly connected to enjoyment, but they are the relationship is not as strong.

Similar to identical to. It is, however, short-lived. The second long-lived One is in the process of taking. Other giving. Dopamine is one of the main ones. Serotonin is another. In-situ gratification and delayed pleasures. Well-being is getting the rest that you require at the appropriate moment, when you are entitled to it.

The pleasure is an element of rewards, however not all rewards are enjoyable. In the case of money, for example.

It is an extrinsic reward. Also, extrinsic reward systems function as motivational magnets which trigger "wanting", but not "liking" reactions once they were obtained. When you receive the extrinsic reward. Then you realize it's not all that great.

There's not a consensus regarding whether pleasure ought to be defined as a feeling or a state of being or an attitude towards the experience or anything else. Yet, that's not the end of the story. Pleasure is an integral part in the philosophical theories that are known as the hedonism. Hedonism involves chasing for pleasure that's quickly rewarding. Self-indulgence.

The most enjoyable and satisfying experiences have to do to satisfying biological urges like food, exercise hygiene, sleep and sexual sex. They are all desires that we have the ability to satisfy with little effort and pressure. But it is contingent on the person and their time of taking place. It is possible to see them as positive or as a negative one. It is a pleasure to appreciate cultural artifacts as well as activities like dancing, music, dance as well as literature can be pleasant.

Instant rewards are a result of having learned something fresh from somebody. We may also learn that we'll enjoy it often. It could be because we wear headphones and can now play our preferred songs. Incredibly, we'll stay away from and gain knowledge from the frustrations you once had after you take a vow to limit the consumption of chemicals, waste time as well as health and material disappearing. Also, we'll change to the latest trends and difficult, yet better and more satisfying in the near future, not even being aware of. As an example, you know the fact that playing video games causes that dopamine boost in your body right now. After you have finished the game, and then look at the amount of time you spent. Then you realize how much time spent and feel depressed and ashamed. Try to fix this problem by... attending fitness classes, helping out around your home, or even learning an important skill that will benefit your future self! This new way of life are painful, and will be viewed as if they were a trap for the eyes. Overall, self-improvement practices which don't please us right now however will serve our health over time. Our brain's neurons produce endorphins and dopamine together with Serotonin and serotonin is a prescribed medication for people suffering from depression so that they feel happier in themselves.

The reason we learn something new is as they fulfill our needs. If we can see, touch the object or smell it that you really like and are enticed by, it is strong to resist. The dopamine receptors in our brains get excited. In response to curiosity, fear or just to make us feel more superior. Our brains love to take in information, and also to discover what's happening on the opposite side of the wall. What will it be as if we are doing drugs, having sexual sex or listening to music or doing a complete exercise routine at the gym. It is through pain that we learn, and we're guaranteed rewards in the moment. In the future, we can reap rewards. or we are learning with exhilaration and adrenaline.

If we are learning something new. We are able to enjoy it sooner rather than later. It also requires less effort to be associated with us. Then we began making patterns in our brains, which were a pleasure to feel. Try it again the next time! "Why should I do it again next time?" It felt great.

If we are doing something that we think is right, it's not always beneficial for next generation. Our minds are constantly telling us that it's better to enjoy the moment and will take us there of, the things we wish for. It is possible that we have mastered something exciting and enjoyable now safe and useful at times. There are certain behaviors that look harmless and not harmful but are slow-burning poisonous to our future self. How come we persist in these same behaviors once we've mastered that we shouldn't be doing the same thing, despite knowing they're harmful? This is a quick reward and doesn't mean we are punished for consequences they can produce. We use social media to get we need social validation and we engage in video games for hours because we are seeking fame and a break from the real world to the virtual. Smoke or eat in order to lessen stress and anxiety. We'll also cover a variety of other habits that we'll discuss in Chapter 4. These habits and routines we make use of or substances we indulge into. They are enjoyable now, but can be dangerous in the future.

It isn't our intention to perform pushups since it's too complicated and we can't imagine the promise of a reward right in the moment. It isn't a good idea to sit and meditate as it's dull and ineffective. We would rather listen to music rather than tidying the bedroom since we're not motivated enough and do not need to do chores.

An effective way to step away from instant gratification is to simply delay the moment and satisfaction. However, we'll discuss the subject later.

The essence of pleasure is that we feel and experience when we are expecting it to be in some way or another. It is a result of the things we take part in, the food and drinks we consume or consume as well as the lessons we are taught and the characters we imitate and seek to imitate. The result isn't genuine happiness or joy in our lives to come. It is appropriate to enjoy a few times. When we do this it is important to keep an educated mind. I'm telling you this because I am aware and believe that knowing precisely the direction you're headed towards is superior to going into the unknown with no thought or a numb mind. However, we'll discuss ways to enjoy instant leisure activities in chapter 8.

:

The pleasure process plays a significant role within our brains. Without it, we won't be able to feel and discover new things, or shift into other feelings like sadness, pain as well as disappointment. other. This is the exact opposite of joy.

The feeling of pleasure or instant satisfaction This is the thing that pleases our hearts right now for a brief duration of duration. Since our brains developed into quick and simple to achieve reward instead of an alternative. Rewards that are delayed and well-deserved. The long-lasting and cherished result of delayed satisfaction.

We are not satisfied in repeating actions time and time again. However, we also need to adapt to change, since we are a species that eats information. It is imperative to understand how certain chemicals, actions as well as emotions affect us. Through the ache of low or extreme effort.

We are taught the behaviors of others and attempt to emulate the behavior of others. We are influenced to emulate the others and do exactly what they do and to be in the instant gratification area. And in the more delayed zone.

Pleasure now might mean harm tomorrow. In addition, the more time we spend with activities that create anxiety or stress now. The less of a good character we will be in the years to come. Simply by comparing our lives to a moment of satisfaction.

Chapter 2: What Is The Difference?

What are the main differences in these? What are the ones that aren't good as well as which are better? The distinctions when discussing the instant and delayed gratifications sound quite obvious. It's true. Two words that are comparable to the two. The words "instant" and "delayed" are similar. It's a good thing because it's going to be right and proper to perform. But if it's delayed, then is hard to do and doesn't merit having to wait for. This is the thing that most of us think about when discussing the issue. But there's more.

Do you know that we can smoke cigarettes to relieve tension over a period of time and smoke once more? It's instant satisfaction.

Do you realize how demotivated and uneasy we are prior to a fitness session?

Then, we're feeling better at yourself? That's delayed gratification.

Things like drinking, smoking and watching interesting content and the habit of eating out or listening to music, using social media to browse, porn, etc. Do you have habits or traits that lead to quick gratification and rewards that are not as long-lasting, and are a threat to our self-esteem for the future. These habits and traits are not only detrimental to the health of us. In terms of social, mental and physically. They also squander lots of money in energy, self-esteem, and even their own. The more we suffer, the more do not think about to suffer. When we are trapped inside a puddle where it becomes more difficult to exit. Each time we seek the instant pleasure.

I am now out in the natural surroundings, doing some exercise by setting small achievable objectives, then long-term goals trying to shed weight using determination and perseverance, stopping drinking or smoking cigarettes meditation, reading books, practicing an ability, working etc. Are delayed gratifications. They are the ones we're uneasy about doing right now. Yet, show us amazing performance in the coming years. These are the results that will strengthen us and assist us.

It is not just about achieving those obvious results of having to resort to a method of delaying gratification we may consider. However, it is also a good idea to increase the patience of those confronting difficult situations, be respectful of ourselves, and look at us as a great person, and receive greater attention and appreciation from other

16

people and even make small adjustments. The first can lead to temporary benefits that are satisfying at the time, but dwindle off fast, while it's a ability to live your life.

Instant gratification occurs the moment you accept the desires of your heart and experience an increase in "happy hormones" like dopamine and endorphins. We generally want items now instead of in the future. The psychological discomfort that comes with denial of self. In terms of evolutionary theory our natural urge is to grab any reward that is available to get it, and restraining this urge is difficult. Evolution has provided humans and other species an intense desire for instant rewards. Infrequent exposure to immediate reward can alter the balance and lead to impulse-driven decisions. This can lead to a variety of mental disorders in humans, like the obesity and addiction. Depression and anxiety. Depression or self-doubt. Delaying gratification is an essential procedure that balances the delay of time and a higher rewards. It's a pain to not enjoy the things we indulge in it's a lie!

Delay gratification refers to refusing to accept the immediate reward hoping that there'll an even greater reward at a later date. It is a result of impulse control people with good concentration on impulse control usually excel in delayed satisfaction. But, delay gratification is another skill one can learn. The delayed gratification trait is linked to being successful in certain ways. But not always is it necessary to wait until we have the things we think are successful within our lives.

The capacity to defergrate can be learned in both adults and children that can help train their brains to be patient. Researchers from University of Rochester University of Rochester wanted to investigate the issue of, "What is delayed gratification?" They then followed up with the well-known Marshmallow Experiment with a new child group and added an interesting twist. The children were divided into two groups prior the test with marshmallows. In the first group, researchers offered rewards such as crayons and stickers. However, they never received the promised rewards. In the second, the promised rewards were fulfilled.

Children in the initial group had difficulty with delayed reward, since they had been taught that that the reward would never happen. There was no reason for them to delay, as the evidence has never provided them with the reason to be able to trust researchers. If you are one of those who is trying to make delayed gratification the norm in our lives There are a number of useful lessons to take from the children. Kids who won the prizes promised taught their minds they were capable of putting off gratification for a while and that delayed pleasure was well worthwhile. This ability to put off pleasure was not born or genetically ordained, but rather an learned behaviour. It is possible to teach your brain to defer satisfaction in many various circumstances.

A refusal to resist any urge to grab the immediate benefit in hopes of receiving higher-valued rewards later on. Our brains can be trained to be patient and wait for a later reward.

In the year 28 years ago, Steve Jobs said what separates individuals who are successful from those which boils down to one simple word. This word was

instant.

Instant Gratification Theory in Psychology

In the midst of instant gratification lies one of the basic motives

human nature: the desire to feel pleasure right now and avoid pain

later. The reason for this is"the pleasure concept. It is also known as the second

commitment. It is the opposite of the instant. Our minds resist the urge to please our

You need to act to be in the present. To ensure a better life for your future. Humans are a definite species.

They are, at the very least in a certain degree, motivated by the need to feel satisfaction.

Today or in the future. It's obvious how we can get instant satisfaction

Compare what delayed gratification offers our. Yet, why do we engage in what we do?

similar bad experiences repeatedly in a state of consciousness or not? A

small reward, or two reasons or for the other, will determine our motives and values.

We will discuss the subject in future chapters. It is important to know

That the activities we engage in as well as indulge in today, can make our lives "happy". Aren't

We should be doing the things that are right and require for our daily life. Drinking alcohol, smoking and video games Netflix or other TV shows eating too much, gossiping, among many others which lead to comfort today. But agony later. Don't be fooled that I am not lying. It is not a good idea to suffer due to it being "fun" and "right" to do it. Then there is the chance to experience delayed satisfaction. Benefits you can enjoy and even pleasant times you are doing these things more and more. You'll begin to appreciate exercising, meditation and reading, working on an ability that can change your life, and on. Then you will begin enjoying yourself more and feel more at peace! If you begin right now is far better than choosing something that isn't happy. It's instant pleasure. A delayed gratification. A far cry from its competitor. Instant gratification. It is a lot better option for health, profitability and sound choice that you can stick with. If it seems difficult and uncomfortable, it's best if... it is if you understand the best way to enhance it. What can we do to use and sustain delayed joy? The topic will be discussed in chapter 4 as well as chapter five.

It is possible to look at the tiny things that make the difference between happiness and pleasure. Also, instant gratification or delayed satisfaction. Outdoor activities are delayed satisfaction over sitting in bed, scrolling through social media, but having no time to work. The habit of making your bed every day before leaving to work or school will result in delayed satisfaction over having your sheets in a mess and tangled. Smiling at your parents and addressing people by giving them a hurt and a warm greeting, rather than ignoring the little habits that can lead to delay in recognition of little by little. This is a result of all the small things we perform or speak. As we continue to repeat or take actions that we're not aware of more likely are we to not start to question the actions we're taking or why we're doing. It will also be simple to overlook the future to make improvements. It is more difficult to look away from our own future self when we keep doing immediate gratification actions and are not mindful of what we do. The more we recognize our actions that can lead us to becoming better or worse potential selves. More likely are we to have the chance of being better than what that we want to become.

Instant gratification feels good right now. It fulfills your needs, whether they are necessary or not right now. This kind of behavior which is a sign of lazyness or low energy, as well as recklessness when seeking a improvement in your self-esteem However, it could degrade the future of your potential. It's what you get today. What you gain right now could turn out to be less later on. This is the wrong direction for you to accomplish anything within your own life. or in your life of someone else.

Delay gratification, or deferred happiness, in the way I define it for long periods of time is not the same as delayed happiness for a long time. It's a kind of experience that is hard, uncomfortable to do now and will be will be beneficial in the near in the future. This might be a sign of an achievement. It is! However, it doesn't need to take place in the future to attain it. Small goals that appear daunting to certain people may cause a massive change on the way we live. While success may typically refer to wealth or money... this doesn't happen most times.

The success of relationship, body and mental well-being, avoiding foolish urges or having the books you enjoy. Can be described as being successful.

and even those little details that are easily visible, but can be a problem for certain people. The little things like making things like making your bed, brushing teeth, or washing up afterwards before someone other person does it. They can have huge effects on your future success.

Chapter 3: How Do We Know It?

In what places do we find immediate happiness and a sense of remorse in our lives and in the lives of other people? Where or in what interaction?

The instant pleasure refers to a brief time of achieving a desire. It can be seen in numerous ways, practices, and products we consume every day. We go through our lives or engage in a way that we do not even realize.

The pleasure of eating junk food is today, but in the future you'll have two extra pounds. Social media allows us to gain an opportunity to be socially accepted by taking our time and creating envy of other people. Video games make players happy however in the end, you do not have anything long-lasting. Instead of having a real experience of adventure and interaction with others instead, you waste your precious time and energy watching an LCD display.

Alcohol and smoking can give your brain a feeling of relaxation. However, it is actually shrinking your lifespan.

Sexual stimulation can give you the impression that you're the only one who has sexual relations, but in reality you are just a sexy jerk who masturbate and does not bother to search for a genuine human being partner. Music, however harmless as it may appear, can be. The release of dopamine puts us in a state of mind for envisioning ourselves as the best version of ourselves. It's fun to gossip about someone however, you do it because of jealousy or self-conscious doubts. The majority of the time, they're not as much of a life ruiner as some. They can be beneficial to our lives in certain instances, provided we recognize and respond to their consequences with a mature sense. In the case of Sex does not ruin a dream when we are able to please the other person and do to be attentive to what other people need. Music that you like when you exercise boosts your the energy level and boosts motivation. Also, eating a little bit of junk food following days of dieting and improvements. These are treats that come following a tiring "day work" but the more you indulge yourself in treats. The less beneficial the effects. This means that there is no need to feel guilt-ridden or stressed when you enjoy the occasional piece of music or sip a glass of wine in a party when you wish to. Don't let the smallest snacks drag you off the track.

This is because it's more convenient to find instant gratification when there is a televisions in our living space and switch to the news. Also, it is easier to look up social media when an Instagram account is always on our pockets every single time. It's easier to purchase unhealthy food items and sugar-laden items when the first thing we encounter when we walk into an establishment are shelves filled with candy. Smoking cigarettes when you are at the bus stop, while someone else is pulling out cigarettes and lighters.

Insane pleasure may be triggered by others too.. We get together with our buddies and a few members decide to eat pizza, and some sweet drinks. There are people who consume alcohol and smoke. We decide to give it a test. After having a good time outdoors and are watching our parents at the television. It can be a reminder of our favourite show. When we speak to one another who bites their lips or simply look away. Since instant gratification does not only provide us with a few short-term reward. It also helps us deal with our issues as well as anxiety.

The obese consume more food items because they feel less than others. They consume more food to relieve tension. The lonely people boogie around due to the fact that they lack someone to connect with. It's a sign of acceptance in society. The more we watch television, the more you feel tired since we are unable to think of something else to do. We play music and then dance in the dark, but we don't have anyone watching. Seriously. What percentage of us are uneasy and uncertain of the opinions of others in the event that we start putting our playlist to the test. However, keeping these patterns and thoughts that are negative inside of us can lead to misfortune as well as pathetic instances. It is better to react immediately to our fears, failures and opinions than to admit that our current behavior will be more detrimental than making changes to better routines. If people ask me what I am not smoking, I just say. "I don't want to, I don't enjoy it."

However, I believe that I need to tell people that smoking does not benefit me but will cause me harm in the coming years.

It is not an exact synonym for being satisfied by something that you have accomplished today or in the future. Humans often get caught up in believing that someone has had a moment of bliss or happiness might mean for other people. We think that they won't be satisfied for ever. A good example would be that those who are successful don't view driving the Ferrari as a quick pleasure. Instead, they see it as something they're happy and proud to have.

Instead, it's the reward that one gets after all the work. "Our emotional brain has a hard time imagining the future, even though our logical brain clearly sees the future consequences of our current actions," this is the way that Laibson states on the campus of Harvard University. "Our emotional brain wants to max out the credit card, order dessert and smoke a cigarette. Our logical brain knows we should save for retirement, go for a jog and quit smoking." Why? because humans did not evolve to be patient and wait for rewards or prize in the future. We were hungry for it immediately. It's still a thrill to feel instant satisfaction in our conversations with people. If someone doesn't seem to be interested when you speak, this could be an indication that you did not provide them with immediate answers to their queries. Also, when we concentrate on one thing, such as video games, for example. Some people may know all about a particular game but others may not understand and get lost in their language. The person who is knowledgeable about video games to look for other people who are knowledgeable about the same topic.

It can happen to us with no thought. Today we understand what an instant pleasure feels like and what it is that makes it so. It can happen to us, and then it comes to us, without us even wanting to do anything about it. We simply stay in the same place until it smacks us. How? We're invited for dinner in someone's house. Following the meal, we are served the second dinner.

Desserts are served. It is possible that they purchased or cooked some high-calorie sugar-laden donuts. There is a trigger that triggers our response to eating too much. A different example could be. On the street, we walk and stumble upon the clothing store. Stopping to take the time to look around, walk in, and later discover that we need to buy a new outfit. We hear music at the distant which entices us to have the look over there.

:

In the present, instant pleasure is ubiquitous as it was in the past. It's more obvious and harder to regulate for our generation. You can just walk outside, or go to the home page on YouTube, Instagram, or Facebook and you'll see immediate-growing content for each individual.. It is everywhere as well as hear and feel it throughout our lives. In a way, it's more than. When we go to the park and see garbage thrown out because the people were not sufficiently disciplined.

Drink and smoke because there is no other way to please ourselves or ease tension. We consume all kinds of sweets because they are everywhere in the retail store's display.

There are many who indulge with instant gratification, such as gaming on video, or enjoying delicious food. We'll give it a trial too. We enter our home and turn the television to one of our relatives' programs, cartoons or even news. Naturally, it's harmful and possibly tempting for certain people.

Even gets there and we don't have to be looked for. It's the other side of the delayed joy. We turn to the television and notice that the channel has an exercise routine. We may also be looking at the work of art that took many years to get to where it is today. The majority of us practice or study how to draw or paint. It is possible to get the sense of competition to be similar to other people.

Chapter 4: What Kills Us?

What exactly is it that makes something enjoyable and relaxing right now more harm in the future? What is the reason to stop these harmful things or behaviors? We do not suffer any punishment for them when we have experienced them, and take part in the same. The truth is. Humans aren't smart We don't really care for the next day We don't wish to believe in the facts often, and we may find ourselves tempted to surrender more than others. Smoking can ease anxiety now. However, it could kill you in the future through the exposure to cancer. Drinking a few beverages every day is not likely to cause any harm right away. However, wait until the pancreatitis or liver begins to show and then subside. Eating more than you normally would not add the excess weight you'd like to keep off of the body currently. Later, the fat may accumulate on certain areas of the body, where it becomes more difficult to remove. Being unable to share equally with a person can result in more. It will also cause you to be an insatiable and ungratifying individual later on. Attending a gathering is a great way to entertain yourself for an hour or so. However, you'll lose time, money and mental energy on the route. Humans make choices that appear without any impact over us today. Yet, it could be a disastrous consequences in the coming years.

Let's take litter for an instance. It is well-known that not placing trash in the right place results in polluted environments and so, why do we continue to litter? We see many trash piles on the roads we walk on and in the fields where in which we plant food in and consume, in parks where we go for a relaxing and reenergizing time at the forest and on the beaches that we refer to as nature's wonders, as well as numerous other locations? What we create pollution and must eliminate is instant satisfaction. Go outside, enter an area of a park, stroll in your community and stay at an airport and look around for litter. Bags of potato chips chocolate boxes, soda cans cigarettes, packages for cigars and bottles of booze. Bags purchased from local fast food chain, etc. and on. Don't keep rubbish in your pocket until you are near a garbage bin or recline point. It makes you less patient and more disciplined. It's what I am sure you may consider. "Patience? How will not throwing away trash and keeping it until I find a bin to throw it make me have any patience and discipline?" The research has proven that people who put off their garbage until they can find the trash container are more organized, accountable, and easy to talk with but as well, they're more thoughtful and admired. The majority of us consume food than we think about and do not consider how we will dispose of our trash that we dispose of. Drinks, food as well as other dopamine-releasing substances do not inspire us to think of food as a source of concern toward our surroundings. It contains nicotine, sugar or ethanol, and can alter our mental state. The nucleus accumbens is which is the part of your brain connected to pleasure, novelty and motivation. It gets too excited, too quickly and cannot be managed. It's not able to concentrate in the present moment in order to let go of anxiety and relax. The feeling is just too intense but also repetitive. familiar.

The act of watching porn and masturbating makes us less confident, embarrassed of our own self, and push our disengagement from social interaction and opportunities to socialize. Particularly by young males, as they feel more weak and less motivated to try things after masturbating. This is despite having a rush of joy. It also causes psychological problems like anxiety, depression and a sense of awkwardness with people we love or would like to bind relationships by. The process takes a significant amount of time trying to find the perfect video to delight you for a few minutes. It will cause you to be miserable all around. The study was done by Jonathan Strum and Dr. Jessica Pyhtila. They discovered shocking findings in relation to the addiction to porn when it was associated with certain groups of individuals. It was discovered that the addiction to porn affects 10% of the adults. About 60% of teenage men. 20 percent of women in their teens. The majority of children who accessed porn websites were between the ages of 10-17 years old. Are you sure that someone who succeeds has more than two hours each day in order to have a t-shirt? Now. Health and energy are the two main things that a person who is successful develops and is focused on. Make these the top priority if you wish to be free or not sex to save your self. The same applies to the sex. However, with sex, there's another aspect. The risk of sex that is not protected increases when you do not take a second thought before making your next step. As your desires will force your to take actions and you'll not like results in the future. However, once you have found your ideal partner, or you become an even better friend. Learn to fulfill the requirements of your loved partner and your own. If you do, then things should go smoothly within your marriage.

Binge eating is often known as compulsive eating. It happens when one eats more food than what they are supposed to, or consumes more food than their stomach is able to handle. Overeating and excessive eating can make someone feel secure, loved and helps calm the person down. Why is this? This is a lot more in connection with emotional trauma, psychological issues that has occurred in the past, fear and doubts about the mental state that create anxiety. Anybody who has been overweight or who was overweight during their past knows precisely the way they feel within their body. We all know how difficult it can be trying to locate the appropriate clothing to dress up and sweating incessantly with no effort, feeling tired and often, feeling uncomfortable even the moment someone mentions that they're overweight, with less control over their anger. True, people who have excess weight due to excessive eating are more aggressive, and also tend to feel more depressed in comparison to people who are not fat! However, this is due to not eating enough. It is because they are prone to medical conditions, liking the way they look and not being confident in their bodies or thinking to this. Binge-eating is a significant disorder that impacts more than 3 million people around all over the world. Binge eating disorder, also known as compulsive food overeating, is a severe eating disorder where people frequently consume excessive portions of food and are in a state of constant hunger. It is common for people to overeat on occasions. While binge eating may sound like something that someone would do without a reason, it's something easier to get rid of than drinking or smoking. It's actually not that easy to overcome the urges of eating too much or obtaining the instant satisfaction of unhealthy food. Obsessive eating has been found as a result of the trauma of childhood as well as abuse to children. insufficient food intake when a person was younger, or receiving the correct diet and consumption they ought to get. If someone experiences discomfort or is uneasy, they may feel they feel a bit tense. Then they turn to excessive eating. It is a serious, easy to see quick satisfaction. A person who isn't eating well could well be tempted to indulge in food over the course of their lives. Why? Since poor nutrition can lead to people eating food that your brain thinks is better tasting rather than being healthier for your body. In the case of binge eating, it can create a great deal of suffering in people's lives and not only psychologically but also physically. It makes you fatter and less attractive. Your clothes don't suit your body anymore, and you feel tired and sweat more easily. Even more irritable, you feel like you are doubting your abilities. Some even take their own lives, and not just due to being overweight. It is because their minds are afflicted by lack of nutrition, and a sense of doubt from their own self or others, simply because they believe they're not worthy and weak.

TV and social media. As social media grew in popularity, TV began falling down little by little. The younger generation, in particular were turning their attention towards a different form of entertaining. You know now what may say about TV. The fact that no one is watching it any more. However and people continue to watch degrading brain content. Also, they waste a significant amount of time as porn searches do. and hours of sleep wasted because they make us stay awake late to watch our preferred television channel, live premiere as well as forcing our minds to search for new and interesting information. What number of hours are you scrolling through the Instagram posting... ? What number of hours have you been able to miss each night in order to catch your favorite TV show ...? How long were you in a solitary room and allow the television or cell phone take over your life? Social media isn't just a way to is a waste of time, but can cause us to miss the opportunities that are available. It can make us feel unhappy, prompts us to take wrong advice and makes us crave things that we'd rather not have.

In particular How many successful individuals have you met on social media who seem to be living a healthier and more respectable life with your own? Do you not feel jealous and even jealous due to their success? What about the many objects like household appliances, clothes or accessories that you don't require but purchased because somebody you follow used the items? Perhaps because advertisements appeared across your screen, and then appeared on our homepages. Perhaps a wrong advice that received from a friend online which you believed was great idea, only later to discover it was an incorrect advice which led to your disappointment and low expectations.

Businesses will pay every cent per pixel they can on their platforms in order to get people more addicted to their services and to make you less happy.

Television isn't that far in relation to social media. We switch from one channel to another on the same channels on television for something that will keep us entertained. We watch comedy programs that bring us to laughter. We can get into Netflix shows for hours, without even realizing. Perhaps the most damaging programs we could watch that make us feel wrong inside of us, and messes up our view of the world is news. It's bad news. Humans love, and I am talking about love. It is thrilling to see disasters and crises and learn about the most recent crime that is broadcast live on the television. It is also important to know how much money or significance someone is to the world. We enjoy political dramas as well as dramatic shows. We enjoy watching mentally degenerated television shows. Also, we like to sit at a table and listen to other people's opinions or experiences. Why?

We want to be aware and we want to know that we're at risk and be prepared for a possible crisis. We are astonished when we hear of the possibility of a crisis in politics, price increase, or a rising number of people unemployed. We are prepared for the worst. We make and plan difficult scenarios to prepare for the tomorrow. We buy extra gas ahead of when it becomes costly. We keep an eye on the news media when they make announcements that are negative. We are able to find jobs that pay better with higher pay when we learn that food prices increase or the percentage of unemployment for a certain area rises.

However, we are also prone to be able to judge people for what they do or say and to play fun with people without considering the implications.

In one instance, I lived in the apartment of one of my aunts resided. They would sit and watch a show in which guests were brought in to talk about banal issues on a variety of banal themes.The participants weren't very trained or displayed a high level of brain function, at the very least. She would then on purpose assess their actions and manner of thinking. She would chuckle and laugh at least a couple of times.

It is present in all of us, more or less. In the form of envy over the things they can do. or because we are annoyed with someone who gets more attention over us. We do not judge them in the open, but we conceal of their insignificant and not worthy of the place.

Then as a very difficult to take pill.

The sound of a giggling gossip is harmless and safe, right? The way it sounds, but it's not. It's a drug as are the other types of immediate pleasure. Why? People love to talk about other people. It is actually fun to learn and learn more about other people as opposed to gossiping about them behind their backs. Are you looking into the specifics, or simply telling a story you heard of somebody? A definition of gossip refers to anyone who divulges personal information regarding others, without letting others be aware. Also, ask if it'll be acceptable to spill the information. When you gossip, it can break your relationship with the person. The loss of boundaries makes other feel that we're untrustworthy. It's the truth. If you keep on circulating untrue or accurate facts about someone public without telling them. and then you disappoint them. It's not fair to break the relationship with them.

The act of gossiping can cut our relationships with people around us and can be an obstacle in forming new ones.

Nicotine and ethanol are the substances we breath in and put through our throats when we wish to enjoy some fun, and ease the tension that comes with. The substances that comprise the solid component of cigarettes are small pieces of solid material, which include phenols nicotine, as well as Naphthalene. Major gasses are carbon monoxide, nitrogen oxides, and anhydrous cyanide. Other liquids comprise formaldehyde, methane and hydrogen,

Ammonia, benzene and Acetone. These are the chemicals that you allow to in your body. Not only the lungs.

Ethanol is also known as ethyl Alcohol. It is made by yeast fermentation of the sugars found in fruit and grains. In the case of wine, it is derived from sugar found in grapes, and vodka is derived with the damsons' sugar or the sour cherries. Ethanol is a chemical used in products for the home that are employed for cleaning. You won't get killed or be injured by drinking cigarettes or drinking alcohol of cigarettes right now. And neither will you the next day. However, the negative effects are as with all the instant pleasures. Then, you can build up until the effects begin becoming apparent. There is a chance that you won't cough and experience pain right now due to smoking. However, when you breathe in smoking, smoke enters the lungs quickly. The blood is then carrying toxic chemicals all over the body. Smoke from tobacco is a source of carbon monoxide which is a dangerous gas, which then depletes oxygen from the blood. The result is that your organs are deprived of the oxygen they require.

Consuming large amounts of alcohol even only a couple of days will cause a build-up of liver fats. This is known as alcoholic fat liver disease. It is the initial stage of the alcoholic fatty liver disorder. Fatigue liver disease is not a cause of no symptoms, however it is a significant warning signal that you're drinking to an unhealthy level. In excess, over time and with no limits.

This is the moment to take the toughest quick pleasure pill to take.

Child raped and abuse . What is the reason why some parents hit their children to show their love or because of out of anger? It's because there are two methods of beating. The first one is where the child is taught as they grow older, and will later be an important life lesson, and they will be grateful and more successful. It is also the one that can transform them into violent and unhappy people after they become adults. Today, no solid parent would beat their child to make fun of them. No rape can be caused by anyone to earn an alleged rapist's title. Yet, I can remember when my mom would spit out her rage at me and my brother every time she did not be smoking something. We would be slapped or yell at us and even threaten us with threats that she would take us to adoption. Naturally, what she said were the words she spoke. Instead, it was the impact that result from smoking no cigarettes for some time or the point where she'll end up with no cigarettes anytime soon. One is always prone to intense anger or frustration whenever they are in someone's presence. Why? It can make the person who doesn't possess an actual "drug" feel better. The effect will occur as the drug begins having less impact, is less used and becoming difficult to get at the time. It will wear off more quickly. It is less used due to various reasons. and to make it more difficult because of the obstacles in order to get their way. The feeling of stress and the pressure of having to do so. There are other methods to let our emotions out and deflect them onto others. We blame others for our actions and making other people feel less than and traumatically affecting people who have nothing to do with contribute to our behavior however, we are in the wrong place in the wrong place at the wrong time. Here's an interesting angle that you can consider. There doesn't need to be someone who takes a particular substance with instant gratification or a enjoyment habit, but never engaging in it in order to ease anxiety and stress. These individuals may have been the victims of those who indulged in instant satisfaction things. An abusive father that beats his kids or a stressed-out brother who is agitated by the absence of sweets or other products, a mother who yells at her children for lack of cigarettes, or a relative who enjoys video games, and displays a lack of respect or anger when ordered to do something positive. The people that raised us weren't required to engage in any of these or overly extreme quick gratification behaviors. It is also possible that they could have suffered abuse by those who were enthralled in immediate satisfaction. Now, they repeat these same errors with their children. Some parents may be suffering from an obsession with lottery games, and get angry when they do not win. Others may want to check out reports or engage in games on their television or yell at people to stop. This kind of behavior can occur even though it's tough to believe they're happening. It's not as shocking as it may seem. Children's abuse can result as a result of a little discontent that's released by the aid of immediate reward. This is because instant gratification is more difficult to attain and is less effective, it is a challenge, or perhaps we want to let it go. The scenarios are similar to the butterfly impact. Now, we take action towards a certain thing and do not think about the consequences. The consequences will later show in the person we might have made some.

Rape is another one which can be traumatic and cause trauma to an individual for life. This can be caused by the pleasure of instantaneous in the present. What triggers someone to engage in sexual sex and rape against the desires of the other? People who are unable to keep themselves in check no longer want immediate pleasure. An urge that cannot be sustained for longer is a flash of joy that explodes. We are frequently influenced by external factors. This kind of action sounds as if a harsh punishment could be imposed. In fact, the next consequences are imposed on those responsible for the offense. Humans can be, at least to in a certain degree, driven by the need to indulge in the pleasures of life. Sometimes, they do it without second thought. With no remorse, an act of quick-thinking and discipline right at the time. People who commit a rape are punished under the laws. They were unable to contain themselves because they felt the pleasure of a moment with negative outcomes. The victims are likely to be affected and will remember the incident with great depth. The initial mental health issue that was examined was posttraumatic stress, a chronic disorder that occurs following a traumatic incident, like a violence.

Disorder (PTSD) disorder (PTSD) is

an extremely troubling

Nearly (40 percent) of victims of rape developed PTSD over their lifetime, and over one-in-ten victims of rape (15 percent) continues to suffer from PTSD today.Rape victim were six times more likely experience PTSD than those who were not the victims of crime. Victims of rape were seven times more likely the current PTSD as those who'd not been the victims of criminality. They will lead the kind of life they don't need to be living. In addition, they are likely to do other inhumane acts throughout their life to ease the burden that has built up and cause harm to themselves or other people. In the end, the butterfly effect begins to take over.

:

True that it isn't going to kill us today or in the future, or cause our bodies harm at the moment. However, later on, the small activities we engage in can expose the sufferer in agony, pain as well as death. In the preceding chapter. The more we push ourselves to do in our lives without even realizing it. The more that we take or indulge in an action, the less effective the result will become. Like a substance that's easy to forget about and accept as harmless. The small side effects can be compounded to create an entire disaster.

The urge to engage in actions that relieve joy, anxiety, and worries, or doubts to feel better right now. Without realizing it could be risky later on. This can create harm to our environment as well as other species.

We indulge in food because we believe that it's a way to escape our previous traumas or poor nutrition.

It is our goal to keep ourselves entertained through porn, and then experience the sensation of what could be real. However that we lose and our energy is the most squandered when we are doing the sexy thing.

We admire others because of their appearance, we don't care for someone else. Sometimes we purchase things to look good and be similar to others since we are unaware of our own situation.

It is easy to get bad advice from the media and presentation.

We talk about other people in order to drink and keep us entertained.

We smoke and drink as we believe it will release dopamine and serotonin However, all we let out are neurons as well as clarity of thought from our minds.

People are abused and pushed to the point that they'll be ruined throughout their lives to a brief feeling of joy. The people who abuse to suffer retribution in the future. It is not just killing us physically but mentally as well as well. And it also causes the death of others who aren't deserving of it.

We are punished for the actions that fast and uncontrollable pleasure makes us perform. It then spreads to another as if it were a bubonic scourge. Abusing, traumatizing the victim, or even raping them could cause them to repeat similar crimes to those they have been through. They will be sanctioned only if they happened to be not at the right time and at the wrong time and in the wrong place. It's not difficult to be the victim of another's wrongdoing. If it happens to us several times then we'll be dragging the same mistake onto other people. This is a butterfly effect. It's a compound effect.

Chapter 5: What's The Reason I Should Be Waiting?

What is the significance of delayed gratification? It's about. Why would anyone wait around to complete something or even to do something instead of now, if you can do it? The fact is, you'll get the outcomes you'd like to see. Being able to wait to a greater reward in the future is a vital ability to have in your life. The ability to delay gratification enables you to make decisions like avoiding huge purchases to fund an escape, not eating food to shed weight or even take on a job that you hate but which helps you deal with finances later. The research shows that delay satisfaction is among the traits that are most beneficial to personal development of people who are successful. Seriously! Someone who has succeeded (not solely with regards to money or possessions.) has waited for a long time to find the right moment that would bring an even more rewarding reward that they have achieved, and are enjoying now. Success doesn't happen easily or over night. A person who desired six-pack abs was aware of the difficulty to achieve it overnight. Anyone who was writing a book had to have ideas and clarity before releasing the work. Someone who was looking for a healthier connection had to wait for a while until they got acquainted with the person more and fulfill their requirements of their partner. They weren't waiting for the reward to arrive to them. They also took action. They fought and slowed down whatever pleasure they may be tempted to indulge in. But they were focused on the primary aspect. It was about getting them the present status they enjoy. You might think you're limiting yourself to in order to accomplish things. But the truth is that it's difficult to attain all that you want or even achieve the item immediately. In reality, instant gratification can be an cause of stress or disappointment. It can also lead to disappointment when you want the most of everything. According to my view I see two possible paths that we could take depending on the situation. One is trying to avoid pain in the present but suffering afterward. There is also a less difficult option of putting off the moment of gratification to achieve a greater goal and a better outcome.

The longer-term objectives are an incentive for those who wait to receive their rewards. Promises and goals are usually the catalysts that motivate us to go even further. It doesn't have to be in the future to inquire why we need to be waiting. This could be something you'd like to accomplish this week. However, they are also likely to give you greater pleasure or alleviate more serious suffering than promises of instant satisfaction. One who is adept at delayed gratification can benefit through the rewards of waiting for a while, such as. The ability to save money for the future, building new abilities faster and more efficiently as well as making relationships with people more easily, resisting urges to indulge in tempting circumstances, valuing the work they do, and making judgments about people, things, or objects with respect to more than one point. However, I believe the primary thing to do is avoid impulsive control.

The ability to control our impulses is what can make us insane and causes us rush towards things we would like. We want something to take place, negative or good. or way that isn't right.

In this case, for instance, someone could be lying to other people to conceal or gain some benefit from them. The other could tell the truth, and not conceal some thing from other people. Someone could get into a fight, and appear angered in their gestures or vocal tones. The other party stays the peace and is reasonable. It is possible to consume more food to avoid stressful circumstances. One can also limit their appetite.

Researchers from Princeton University from New Jersey. There are two regions that make up the brain. One which is connected to emotions, and another associated with abstract thinking. You may have noticed it is the emotional component of the brain is responsive to instant satisfaction. If you are presented with the option of the cake right now or later broccoli that part of your brain prompts your to pick the cake. Why? Your Brain Prioritizes Instant Gratification Over Long-Term Goals? You are aware of your responsibilities, yet you continue to indulge in impulsive control. Most of the time it is the case that the abstract and logical part of the brain may not be sufficient to motivate you, as is that of the emotional. The rational part of your brain however, is trying to convince your. It could suggest that eating broccoli is good for long-term health and you don't require this chocolate cake. It's not always successful, and it's hard to beat your emotional side of your brain. The logic and emotion-based areas of your brain remain engaging in an argument in an attempt to demonstrate what you need to know about an option instead of one.

Which portion of our brain will win ultimately? It is contingent on the circumstances. Researchers concluded that impulsive actions occur in situations where the emotional portion of our brain triumphs over the rational one. Why? It is because these people do not have self-control, are prone to greater impulsiveness in their lives and being in poor conditions and are surrounded by influences.

The successful people who have reached their current position because they waited. Discipline and time management and keeping a consistent attitude. If you wish to be successful in your daily life, you must wait or delay rewards, then keep working on it continuously. Naturally, you can't simply sit and expect success to happen it is necessary to make the effort. Because time, consistency and intelligent choices and actions = the success you've always wished to accomplish. A person who worked out to reduce weight and strengthen muscles consistently worked out. Anyone who wants to gain recognition and to sell their paintings, was waiting for an opportunity to kept up their vigilance. Similar to increasing their income. Millionaires waited to find the right moment. In the meantime, they accumulated all the knowledge they could. In the words of Adam Smith once said.

"The world's most successful people didn't wait for someone else to pick them, but instead, they picked themselves."

Waiting requires self-discipline. It is one of the traits we must develop and master. To be more self-controlled you have to be willing to put in the difficult work whenever we aren't feeling like doing it. Even when we fall short and discover that joy isn't always easy We must continue and improve. Discipline is a trait that's extremely easy to attain. In the following chapter, we'll learn more about discipline and how it may impact our lives. However, I would like to discuss the factors that make us successful within our daily life.

I'll repeat it a few times again.

Time +

Consistency +

Innovative choices and action = successful.

The cultural norms that surround us urge us to look for temporary solutions with Band-Aids and to soothe us. Basically doing whatever is necessary to alleviate our pain today. Don't wait around or perform a lot of effort. It is evident on evenings when we indulge in unhealthy food, instead of losing weight. Poor compulsive control. The couch is occupied all day playing video games, instead of working. It's a stupid way to spend all entire day. Imagine being a wealthy individual instead of taking risks and learning things that can be profitable. Inconsistent behavior and inconsistent behaviour. Our lives are now in which it's easy to lie on the couch and enjoy yourself to have a quick cigar or drink, as well as browsing social media. Instead of making the decision to put these ways of life, and instead seeking out new and excellent alternatives. A few people aren't convinced of how important it is to be patient when things get tough or working toward a target that they would like to drop the pounds now in the quickest method. and would prefer to buy the newest, most powerful cellphone rather than invest in an the investment they'll make in their business. Also, they would rather play Netflix instead of exercising just 10 minutes. It is common to make life decisions based on how we will avoid suffering now, but by doing this, we do not realize that the route of delaying satisfaction is often the best solution to our issues lie.

If someone is so close to getting the reward they desire, their emotional mind takes over. For instance, if you see a chocolate cake is looking right at you, it become clearer about the brain's part that is winning. But. If you stay on track and learn to teach yourself the right principles, it are beneficial to your future. If that identical piece of cake looks at you. You can imagine what would occur to your future self should you decide to eat the cake. Similar principle applies to any other substance or action. However, at a minimum it is important to tell ourselves that we will at the very least, put some effort in analyzing the potential consequences for our future self when we take certain actions or behave in a negative manner. The reason we are waiting for so long before putting in the effort and consistency.

If we're looking for the success we're hoping for is often the one you least think to be. It's also the most difficult to reach. Perhaps you'd like to shed the excess weight you've put on your waist however, you're not sure what you can do or what time it's going to be. And what is it that makes a good person who waited patiently for their results and was aware of the steps to take? A lot of people who are as normal as they look will tell you that determination, discipline and self-maintenance contributed to loss of weight. But, the majority of people have a different opinion, and the majority of people would disagree with your opinion on this. The perseverance, self-control as well as a surge of enthusiasm led to the loss of weight for someone. They'll fade away only to come back in the event that we require the same thing. This is the suggestion I'd like to give to you.

Do not think too much about your time spent making yourself better, and don't get discouraged when you do not see what you want to see. This is applicable to every possible achievement you can think of as being feasible. Perhaps, saving money? Put your money aside to save for the future, with no knowledge of how much you've saved, or without thinking about the amount you have did save. Are you looking to lose weight and build muscle? Keep your goal in mind and work out in the way you believe is best for you until you achieve the results that you've always wanted. Spiritual wellness? You should spend your time and energy contemplating ways to not leave you feeling exhausted or bored.

Instead of being seem so simple and bold. Create it in a relaxed way and with control. Don't keep track of every penny, calorie and moment you've had. Place them in your personal control. In the end, if you aren't in control of your own life somebody else or something can do it. Don't you want to live a life that is controlled.

:

The idea of waiting for a delayed reward may appear to be a difficult thing to accomplish. But, your amazing results will be worth each second of the decisions made, ideas, and efforts you put in.

As a result of delayed reward, it is not just a long-lasting reward, but also the acceptance. You also learn to be more patient and shrewd under pressure, and enjoy more self-esteem. Also, self-control in stressful scenarios.

Some people avoid delay-gratification due to the fact that they are not well-organized enough. They live living in an age that our values and the technology allows us to get what we want and without having to wait or putting in lots of effort. We live in a negative surroundings, or in the presence of undesirable people who affect our lives and form our lives. The smallest change in the passage of time, wise decisions, consistent actions and choices could be ineffective for someone trying to make a change that is going on in their lives, and later abandons the effort. However, it is crucial for a prosperous individual.

The waiting for you to learn the best way to defer any rewards today isn't the same thing as being lazy, indifferent or not achieving anything. It's a valuable life skill that could improve and utilize to live our lives to the best date and at the right time. Learning to utilize the timing with a sense of consistency can be an important life skill.

Instead of feeling anxious and having bad management, take control of your personal daily life. Be a team when you commit to actions that ensure you are in the correct direction for what you want to accomplish. Do not be overwhelmed by concerns or issues. Be aware and in charge of your cravings and waiting.

Chapter 6: What Can We Do To Make Improvements?

In chapter 2 we've covered as well as chapter 5 a few aspects of the advantages of utilizing a delay in reward over instant reward. However, what we must be asking ourselves is how can we stay away from temptation and remain cognizant of our actions and the way we behave. There are a variety of ways to getting rid of bad practices and accepting different ones. What can you do to help your brain relax and make wise choice for delayed gratification. Although we're able to use the rational aspect of our brains to aid us in our decisions but we could easily get into decisions that aren't beneficial to the long-term interest of our family.

An habit tracker can be useful for those who want to make a commitment to what we'd like in our lives. You can also stick notes that you've written about what you plan to accomplish for the day. It should be written in a happy manner to do your best and not with shame after you indulged in the pleasure of instant enjoyment.

In my case, for example created the calendar, and put it to the door of my bedroom. Then I wrote on it the things I do, and plan to do. I listed my workout schedule and meditate, go to the bed, brush my teeth at 8 hours a evening and on. If I accomplish things that are written down in my calendar, I make a note of it using a checkmark and mark things I did not commit to by marking it with an x. Try writing the date for tomorrow. on a sheet of paper, your smartphone, or desktop. creating it into your wallpaper can ensure that you are committed to the idea you wrote down to do. Why? We write it down using our hands or if we do not take a vow to the words we did. We are embarrassed of ourselves. We feel like we've lied to us.

Be constantly telling yourself what can expect if you take something that is either good or bad outcomes can be a good habit-tracking and commitment solution. You will also make impressive progress to take note of and celebrate. The sign of deferred gratification can be achieved by affirming you

"I am not going to do that." or "I will get to do it!" This gives you the honesty and drive you have for committing to your daily tracking routines.

Here are four strategies that you can apply to help you live your day.

1. Be aware of your surroundings as well as surround yourself like-minded people. I've observed that cravings arise mostly

when we view the smell, taste or talk to these people. There are sweets and desserts at the table, and then hide healthy foods from view in the back of our refrigerator. It's much easier to indulge in unhealthy foods that causes weight gain and be embarrassed afterwards. This method is employed by every major supermarket chain. In small, corner-sized alimentation shops. The majority of us will buy things that are first our sights, rather than the reason in the back. Most likely, the product we choose looks good or has a unique look. However, put nutritious food in a bowl at the table, and be clear about it. How come we choose to eat the food we have in front of us instead of looking for an alternative that is healthier? It's simpler for our brains to think this way and also less stressful with regards to preparing the food we need.

Smoke more and consume more alcohol when we are around people who have the same habit. However, separating ourselves in a group of people such as these, we can cut down consumption of alcohol and nicotine significantly.

It is common for us to scream more often when we spend a lot of hours in bed with nothing to be doing. There are devices, and an internet access that keep ourselves "entertained" for a long duration. There is a feeling of being released, and experience something that sounds like joy as well as achieving our objectives. In reality, we create our own mental abyss. Do you want to increase your muscle mass and improve your fitness? Notes are a great way to remind yourself that you'll exercise this morning in the exact time and place you'd like to. I've done this more than I remember, and still get asked why I am so motivated to work out. Additionally, having a person who is motivating your motivation to exercise. You want someone to portray, admire or construct the exact physique following. Bring us motivation and energy. It is commonplace to see runners running every day to increase their endurance and resistance. On our own, we are likely to follow in their footsteps. If we observe people in the gym who are doing heavier lifting than we then we will likely strive to be better than them when it comes to lifting weights.

Do you want to write your own book But the noise in your home distract you? Choose a peaceful place to take a trip there to work on your novel. The library or cafe, or even visiting someone else's home for a moment of calm and motivation will work.

It's not all about meeting new people or creating the right environment. Controlling your environment is also helpful for those who want to accomplish some important objective. If, for instance, I'm planning to meditate, I'll clean the room prior to beginning. It calms my mind and allows me to be able to complete no more work once I'm finished meditation. If I decide paint, I ensure that I do not make a mess when I'm done. I tidy up the water jar, paint containers and the brushes to make them easily accessible moment next time. If I decide to sit down and read. I'll ensure it is near me and readily accessible as I lie on my the bed.

Being aware of your surroundings and managing it is essential in deciding to defer your pleasure. There is a strong urge to sip a glass of beer when you see your friends drinking the drink. It's difficult to convince yourself to go on an outing if we fail to locate our running shoes, and don't enjoy the activity. It's impossible to be productive when we've got on our desks the gaming console that will keep us occupied throughout the course of our day. Therefore, a suitable environment is necessary for making a difference.

2. Provide for basic necessities.

If possible, discover ways to engage the emotions of your brain. In the event that your brain seems to be continually pushing you to do some thing, it could indicate the level of energy you have.

Are you exhausted? You can take a nap or some rest prior to your next exercise. Do you have a stomach ache? Take balanced meals throughout the day and avoid fast food and junk foods. Feeling stressed? Note down the things that frustrate you or get rid of your negative thoughts through exercise. Are you tired of reading too many books or feeling obligated to read? Take a moment to relax and pay attention to what the author would like to convey instead of exceeding your limit too much. If you're not being properly taken care of the mood can drop and your thinking skills get worse. It's why we find ourselves wanting to quit after a hard work out, writing a book or gaining confidence in the skills we'll need in the future. We exhaust ourselves without realizing, and we take excessive action even which we ought not to. Being lazy or not taking a different action in lieu of what you initially planned can be productive in the long run for a delay of satisfaction, so long as it's effortless and does not frustrate your.

3. We get our emotions from people around us. It is said that surrounding us with our surroundings and individuals who are for our benefit is important. However, they do not require any communication with us. Why? because when a person who is disciplined observes someone else who has achieved an achievement in their lives and strives to attain the same level of achievement, if not even greater. The emotions we feel can override our logic deductive abilities. possess. When you next see people doing something you would like to do. Remember to emulate the person you admire. Did you see someone looking in good shape, and having fun with other people? Make an effort to replicate one of their achievements. Have you heard someone read out loud on a page before a crowd in complete confidence? Be determined

to improve your speaking and reading abilities. Learn from others when you are determined to create a habit and connect it to an emotion. Consider that you're sharing an area with someone who whom you have never met and they did not meet either of you. You both have one bed each to sleep on. Based on your level of discipline and the awareness that you won't be evaluated in the beginning. A person might make the bed early in the morning but the other one will not. The bed is only a few days later when that the other one decides to make the bed, and to be a little more than the one who completed your bed. Humans are drawn to imitate the actions of others. Particularly, the methods used by others to achieve success.

4. Do it now. Do not do something you'll regret in the future. There are people

I've heard who are able to commit to the things they want to do by declaring that they will not or do it. I tell myself I'll perform more push-ups or crunches if I'm feeling exhausted or disoriented It is effective! It may seem unprofitable and pointless, but it really works! The act of telling yourself what to take action and not can be very helpful when you want to enhance some thing. Why? What exactly is it?

The brain is more conscious about the results of your actions prior to when you take them, or afterwards. If you say out loud or in your mind what you expect to gain by committing to a particular action. It will be viewed as a judgement by yourself in the event that you do not take the pledge that you made about what that you'd perform. You will also become anxiety-ridden and nervous if aren't able to commit to the things you planned to do the first time. Doubting yourself is a bad thing. It is the reason we should affirm what we are going to receive, whether bad or positive. We'll be more conscious of our actions and promises.

It's possible that a habit tracker sounds too stressful, and you'll likely give up after a few times.

What are we able to doing and document the things we have done and those we didn't do? Create a system that is easy and fun.

I mentioned that managing your environment, and remaining with an environment who are most compatible with you is sufficient.

But! There is a chance that you will not be reading each night before going to bed, or meditate on a daily basis. This is fine. If. you only miss one time! If you keep trying to not make it to more than once. It is easy to give up. It's not my intention to skip the day or even take a day away from writing exercising, doing your workout, or working on your skill, but then do it and again. No! It's about getting back to your original location in the quickest time possible.

:

Habit trackers and commitment devices are fantastic when we wish keep a new habit as well as something that will comfort us to come back to. For instance... recording your plans for tomorrow. Notes you've written and making a commitment to them whenever you're going and then referring to the notes. Also, not putting away factors that can help you yield a significant result. or simply telling yourself about what could happen to you in the future in the event that you perform the actions you've planned for.

Controlling your surroundings and surrounding yourself with people who you'd like to be around confront problems can be more helpful than we think. The less friction we experience, the more peace we can feel with our surroundings and other people. We will see more positive results. achieve later on.

Don't keep away healthy foods we eat when we wish to shed weight, and to stop purchasing unhealthy food items by not taking our wallets out in order to save cash. Making a habit of sleeping earlier and putting away all distractions, and clearing our thoughts by exercising for just 5 minutes prior to bedtime can yield amazing results in the future.

An habit tracker could be one that is simple to acquire and utilize, fun, and not considered something to do. It is easier to become attached to an item that is simple and fun to be committed to. The simpler and more reliable it is to use a habit tracker, more often we'll utilize it and be committed to it.

Chapter 7: Discipline, Containing Yourself.

Mastering self-control can be a struggle. It's true that even understanding the ways to improve discipline in an apprentice can be difficult! Being someone who chooses to engage in bad behavior whether consciously or not, may be difficult, it is certainly not insurmountable. In my case, for example, had a difficult time to complete daily chores. In addition, I didn't have the motivation to complete anything for the majority of my time.

There's good news although it might appear as if you have none of the control in your life, the truth is you have control over your life. But you may not realize this but. What you have to learn is some strategies for self-control. In fact, it's just some guidelines to get you in the right direction in the direction of altering your lifestyle. For you to escape immediate pleasure, and to reap slow but steady gains of delayed satisfaction.

Self-discipline is among the skills that requires constant development and practice, like any other skill that requires time to grow. If you are willing to practice, you will discover ways to develop your self-discipline. However, first let's look deep into self-discipline. Self discipline refers to the capacity to manage your behavior, emotions and thoughts. If you are concerned about the loss of weight, and you are efficient, you're not going to allow thoughts of slackness and unambitious thoughts linger on your mind. It is your goal to eliminate them through telling yourself what you want to do about the future to see what's going to occur.

If you are overindulging in food more than you ought to. If you aren't sure what is the best thing for you You will be thinking carefully before committing to overeating or eating food. Again. Be aware of the results you'll face if you go through the negative things, and the better ones. Anyone who is successful at whatever area you consider their choices. It could lead them to fall. or directly towards their goals.

These are a few tips that you can implement in your everyday life to get a greater delay in your reward.

1 . Begin by counting down. Then, take action.

If you're struggling to get motivated One way to get motivated is to use a countdown clock and then get moving. You can then force yourself into doing what you're doing. The simple countdown may aid in putting you in the correct mental frame to be motivated. Maybe you'd prefer to incorporate it into other things. Take for example, three deep breaths, clenching your knuckles or twisting your neck to avoid becoming motivated before you do any other activity. Are you not feeling up to doing another set of push-ups? Three deep breaths before doing another set. Are you afraid to answer a call? Make sure you twist your neck at least two times before you answer. It's best to count your time prior to doing things when you aren't feeling inspired to complete something. Sometimes, all that is needed is a bit of motivation to move that step.

2. Set your goals in a place where they are visible every day. Even the small ones. Set as many goals as you'd like to achieve. Small, medium and huge ones. They should be put on the ground where

you will observe them daily prior to completing the task. Overlook them with anger and determination. Do not hide them. Try to remember that you've got targets to meet. Write goals down and place them somewhere you'll be capable of seeing them may be found in numerous spots. The wallpaper on your phone can be an incentive to remember your goals. Put it down on your desk.

3 . Remember why you began.

In all of the self-discipline suggestions here, this will help keep you up when things get tough. Maintain your ultimate objective in your mind and don't allow yourself to get lost in the reasons you began. If life is to the limit, don't let it stop you. Try to push harder by thinking of the reason you began. Finding a reason to continue moving is essential. This is why it's important to remind yourself of the reason you got started. Why didn't you throw up, take the walk, spend less or even save money.

4 . Find someone who will make you accountable.

There is a lower chance that you will be a cheater If someone else is watching. What's the matter? Can someone else assist me continue? You can do it without being conscious of it. We'd like to impress the most impressive on our very first day at the at work. We'd like to tidy up the home whenever someone is coming to visit us. We'd like to show our guests that we are able to save the money. Why? We do not want to be as weak, insignificant, or unmotivated to other people. This can serve to help you to reap the benefits of a delayed process. Keep your close friends around your family members, you or colleagues as people whom you wouldn't wish to fail to please. It doesn't have to be a requirement for them to be your closest friends however, they should be someone you think about never lying with or fail to disappoint.

5 . Recognize your weak points. If you're looking to learn how to manage your self-discipline be proactive in tackling the weaknesses you have. Find out how easily you fall and then figure out how you can stop it from occurring. As an example, you should know what time to halt when the you are under pressure. Do not starve yourself lose weight. Also, do not overload your brain while studying a new language avoid working too much for your low earnings.

Another method to determine the weaknesses of your system is to consider timing and where you are. If you're unable to purchase the item you'd like this month. It is likely that next month you'll have the money to buy it. Also, if you're planning to create a novel with a tangled family. This is not ideal for the task you're thinking of. Being aware of the timing and best location can help our lives more than we imagine.

6. Do the thing. Staying away from instant satisfaction is simple. There is no need to eat too much or smoke, drink or play video games or waste any more of the earth's space. Change something about your daily life. Even if only for a short time, or just 1% improvement to the thing you're working on. Begin by telling yourself that is easy. How? Simply tell yourself to get rid of that negative, influential side of you. Get to work. There are two sides to this. It's the one that is lazy. It's also efficient. If your lazy, unreliable, harmful part of yourself

comes into. The productive, hopeful and recognizable part is the one that needs to get out. You have a chance of getting it done, and of going from being unproductive to becoming efficient. If you're feeling up over not being reading... since... this is exactly the way your toxic side is going to react. Don't make the same mistake since... this isn't even clear purpose. It's lazy and useless is a waste of your time, space and money. The good thing about you, the part that recognizes the value of things and thinks differently is able to take action based on clear reasoning and comprehension.

These are just examples of things that could help someone begin to develop the level of discipline. We can also develop it by doing the difficult task even when we don't feel or want to. The reason I say this is because our brains search for comfort continuously and in a constant manner. How? Do you remember the time when you wanted to get up and get your work done? You would say to your self "I will do it later" and an hour or even two hours, would go in silence without any action. "Wait? Isn't this the fourth method of how to improve on delayed gratification? " It's not really. Let me explain it. If we are looking to accomplish something, we do it. For example, ask someone out. It is a great idea be able to establish a connection with the person. However, we receive signals from our brains about not contacting that person. Why? We all know that our brains want comfort instantaneously and in constant fashion. When we aren't ready to rise from the comfort of our sofas. or when we aren't ready to do for an additional 5 minutes. or finish a task that is important. Why?

We are able to do it more easily, not only physically, to lie on the floor and do nothing. Also, psychologically. This puts us into an immediate gratification path. A lower level of discipline means more enjoyment in a single moment. A lower level of discipline will bring you more immediate pleasure.

When we are faced with the thought that we are not doing something such as saying something or performing actions on a regular basis. This is the time for us to reaffirm our commitment to doing the task that appears to be hard. Do you feel not inclined to go for the walk? Let your mind stop and do your heart. Do you feel like giving up practicing your guitar? You can remind yourself of what you were doing when you started, and then snap away from procrastination. Do you find yourself unable to resist the temptation to not eat too much? Consider the way you'll look when you eat too much. Simply tell your brain stop since our brains fool us into looking for the comfort of. Being aware of what is right and adhering to taking the correct actions. It's essential.

Discipline doesn't come only through the words you say to yourself. It can also be derived from the environment, and even past events. Let me explain. An overweight person may find themselves in a state of fear and shame to be mocked every time someone mentions they're fat. By being ridiculed. People will indulge in more to avoid a humiliating event. A different example would be when smokers are in a place in which smoking is prevalent and they are free to do so. In the park, they are and observe others smoking. They are in a park and there is no one. The park will be associated as a smoking place. When we go to the home of a close friend and find them playing games that we would like to. We will then consider visiting their house. The thought will come up prior to getting there to play games like they did the last time. What does all connection have with discipline, in the first place? It is possible to stay away from temptations during that particular time and location, isn't it? Yes! There is a chance that a few individuals won't eat too much when they're being ridiculed smoking cigarettes at a park, or play video games when they are at friends' homes and witness the kids having fun. In many instances, people are motivated by things, places and times of the past. It's not just about people or the arrangements . Therefore, it's often simple to indulge in whatever you like whenever we go to a location which reminds us of previous desire. It can be very simple to mark a boundary, and adhere to the path that you've drawn not to do the things that a location or an event inspires in us.

Discipline can be described as a or a level. More you perform the activities you're not interested in doing, or feel slow, or when you're in situations that are difficult to overcome. You don't have to do anything to change it. The less disciplined you be, the more unruly you will. The more you count down when confronted with stressful situations can help relieve tension. Making things visible and easily identifying your objectives can be another way to do this. When you are reminded of the reasons why began to follow your objectives.

The presence of someone who is watching your shoulders and make you conscious of your choices acts as a pacing device.

Being aware of your weaknesses and understand where to begin and the best place to begin is a crucial aspect.

Just do it. Take action now, in the way your intuition advises you to. If you do not take advantage of the opportunity to hear your own brain, then you are missing the positive aspect of the experience will be lost. You allow your guard to fall down to let the negative portion of yourself grow larger and more powerful.

Self-control is the key to discipline. When we find ourselves within a situation that has influenced us to commit undesirable things, it is important to be able to resist temptations of the earlier. If we encounter certain occasions where our old ways have been shining.

Chapter 8: What To Do When You Want To Be Indulgent.

In our daily lives, we'll indulge with the pleasure of instantaneous enjoyment. At times, we don't even realize or for a long time. The goal of perfection is not something we can attain and therefore, it is not necessary for an ideal life. This is due to not being exhausted when trying to attain excellence, of not transforming into better than who that we could be, and not recognizing ourselves as in the ways we do not want to become. There are times that instant happiness can help. In the end, life is supposed to be a pleasure, and perhaps not wasted. Take a take a look at what I'm trying to talk about .Remember that, in the end, you shouldn't keep everything inside and try to keep our minds. Our emotions are there to be aware of and deal even when it leads us to the edge of instant happiness. However, I believe that the feelings that lead us to the instant pleasure and ruining our lives little by little are the feelings that the irrational side of us has been performing. Our brain that's not sure of what's best for us, and is prone to using whatever comforts it can to keep going. It is possible to control the sudden emotion which can lead us to seek out instant pleasure. Think logically, and think ahead of any release method or move before diving directly into these feelings. We can't stop them at any moment and anyplace. The distractions and imbalances will make them and eventually you will become a victim. Then we'll become more aware of our actions and will realize that we gained from them. Stress, a feeling of anxiety could kill us and even rotten us if we do not manage the issue in a responsible manner. It is based on where you're located. it is not possible to release stress there. Also, depending on who you're together, you cannot allow it to be released before them, either. When I'm feeling stressed, I workout, clench my teeth, and press more. When I'm sad, I make a list of my goals concentrate on something that will be profitable. Also, when I realise that I have no any control over my actions or what I'm doing but I am unable to think. I try to relax with a few breaths, and waiting few minutes.

Music, for example. James clear, who is the creator of Atomic Habits said in his writing that he had been disqualified from rejoining the team and was there on the court for the second time. After recovering of a serious accident, it was more than 6 months to heal. He'd find himself weeping in his car seeking a song to let go of the stress and anger of what people told him. What made him turn to the radio in his vehicle and look for a tune to help him calm at what appeared to be difficult times for him in the past? What happens when a person is working out. They turn on their favourite music and begin to work out in order to improve their body. Also, when doing things that are monotonous and requires lots of time. We tune into music, or radios from several postcast channels. Why? Because it's dull, we lose motivation and focus whenever we are doing the same thing over and over again and it takes an enormous amount of time. I began with music since it's not nearly as hazardous like other instant-gratification actions. It also helps us, even if we eventually become bored, or switch to another technique. But what about different activities? We are aware that these activities are harmful and can cause pain to the future. When we gossip and robbing others of us, there is nothing good that is going to come from this, so why do continue to do it? Like I said earlier in the first chapter Chapter. The pursuit of perfection will always be there. I do not want to demoralize anyone and put them in the impression that they are in a state of despair or that they aren't doing the right actions, but it is inevitable that we be prone to some instant pleasure things. This is why it's important to take a step back and think about what's coming for us in the near future. When we are in the immediate gratification zone. It is important to go in using an adult mindset. with a shrewd and organised views of time. You don't want to get there and discover yourself after years of enjoying the immediate pleasure, but forgetting about the longer-lasting joy. If we're smoking, gaming and eating food that isn't healthy, or whatever else immediate gratifications we can get. Make sure you have an adult mind. It is more likely that you will leave and then be aware of the results you're doing and you will not be doing them frequently as often as you did in the past. Stand up with your hands and declare that you're likely to spend your time, and neglect assets to get an instant thrill. Check yourself looking in the mirror, and state you are aware of what are getting when you engage in instant pleasure. Take note of the actions you take in the event that you realize they may take you down a different direction than what you're on before committing to. The next time you are struggling to end something that gives you instant satisfaction. Then you realize that you are having to do it less frequently as you did in the past and until you feel your life miserable. your daily life. Think with an adult mind. Consider what the results could be for the future version. Imagine the amount of amount of time that you'll lose if you play another game on video, think of the person you will be in the future as you eat junk foods, and think about your character when dining with someone and are chatting with someone drinking a glass of wine with smoking your cigar. Delay. Instead of responding to the impulse right away when it occurs, with no awareness in your body. You shouldn't take action immediately. Give yourself some time between the desire and the action. Your heart rate will get back to normal. Your breathing gets a little deeper. Relieve yourself. In essence, relax and consider any foolish decisions you'll regret in the near future.

It's like having a child. As much freedom you offer them, the bigger an experience they'll have as they are older. It is essential to do this even when you are caught in situations that are tempting, with in a limited amount of time or forced to do so. Maintain your focus and discipline in your mind. However, here's a one we can consider asking ourself. You, whatever you're called. You should you ask yourself. "What activity gives me both instant gratification and delayed gratification?"

Once you've discovered this solution, you'll have the pleasure and gain in the near future through immediate pleasure. As an example, I love to listen to my preferred music and feel pumped. However, I also love to experience pain in my body due to the specific exercise I perform and the energy it brings me. Also, I enjoy listening to what others might call "boring and useless" podcasts as I paint. There is always ways to adjust to both delayed and instant pleasures in one go or within a reasonable distance. If the accuracy of this could be addressed this would be like an ultimate goal, a most important thing you can do which is something you feel good about in the present, yet is difficult or uncomfortable. However, it makes your feel better in the future. There's a good chance that one might be wondering how to avoid putting the garbage at the correct place when enjoying their favourite food, or working on their internet venture in a park lifting weights, or tossing the garbage wherever they'd like to. It's different from performing a foolish act when you are working towards a more successful future.

Chapter 9: Time Of Entitlement

Have you ever had to be in knee-deep water taking care of your kids as they browse through their mobiles, unintentionally to the back pain that you suffer in order to clean up the mess they leave behind? If so, then you're one of those who are a victim to the system which allows kids and teens to be so entitled they aren't even willing assistance to their parents that are getting old in the home. Although it's easy to sit and accuse this person without a face named society for their children's mishaps It is your obligation to try your best in order to aid those who need help. For this to be done, we need to comprehend the idea of entitlement. The concept of entitlement can be described by the term "an unrealistic, unmerited, or inappropriate expectation of favorable living conditions and favorable treatment at the hands of others" (Porter 2021). The goal is to investigate and examine both the previous as well as the present reasons for the notion of entitlement across society in order we can stop the negative effects it causes on children of today. Let's examine the present state of entitlement, and consider what been the cause of its apex.

People are becoming increasingly irritable due to the growth of technology such as the internet. The same is true for children, who have their attention fixed on smartphones, which could do almost anything with the touch of one button. The result is that they eventually become bored with things that take more than a couple of seconds. TikTok videos are usually around a minute in length for an explanation. Attention spans are decreasing that means that your children won't be able to finish any project you assign them, especially if it doesn't come with the promise of instant rewards. With attention spans getting smaller and smaller and shorter, how do we demand someone to do the job they have or look after children or animals when they quickly get bored? Although these children haven't yet matured but I'm wondering what their limited attention spans could affect the aspects of our lives that need long hours of effort and time. It is likely that if they cannot view a commercial for 5 minutes prior to watching a show on TV and they won't have the ability to cook dinner in 45 minutes. My kid would have been watching YouTube for hours If I let him however, that's not the only thing which will be affected by the short attention durations. What is the future of literature or art? What will be the next generation of writers or artists to draw or write for the current generation, even if they're not capable of focusing for more than 5 minutes? These activities relieve stress and tension. However, the younger generation won't bother due to the time it takes. It is my belief that this could cause general discontent; perhaps it'll be referred to as "The Great Depression Part Two."

Shows on reality television are detrimental to young people. The shows like Keeping Up With the Kardashians, The Bachelor, and Too Hot To Handle are teaching youngsters that it's OK to be arrogant and entitled. They also teach unattainable body standards that could be harmful to your child's emotional health, self-esteem as well as body image. The shows mentioned above are a few examples of the foundations of the culture of eating disorders, which has been embraced throughout popular culture for a long period. Check out runway models who appear to be starving to conform to the way we think women should dress. People on these shows evidently display these behaviours in order to create captivating content that is shocking to their viewers and makes kids believe it's okay to be this way. I've seen real fights with siblings on the shows and also people who have mentalities that tell them they're better than others because they're beautiful or have a lot of money. This not only encourages the narcissistic, entitled lifestyle however, these shows often depict alcohol-related abuse and a manner that is believed to make it a normal thing, which is one that I find a major pet peeve in our culture. There is nothing wrong with having some drinks in order to let off steam However, some youngsters today will be drinking for extended periods of time and then end up in hospital.

Technology is again having influence on every aspect of our lives. The latest form of parenting known in the media as "iPad parenting" has enabled an increase in the number of spoiled kids who have a tendency to throw tantrums. Particularly parents, who are young and bustling parents have been recognized for giving their children devices from an early time to help them calm down while they're too busy dealing with tantrums. I get it. I don't like screaming children equally as any other individual, however this impacts children over the long term and only makes them more likely to continue behaving in this way. Children's devices exposes them to the risky waters of internet (parental control isn't sufficient for many applications) However, it also reinforces the notion that, if they start to cry and cry, they'll be given an electronic device that they can play with. This is basically rewarding the child who is crying and consequently, they'll cry more. The child learns through trial and error but not succeeding. If they attempt to cry in order in an attempt to gain their attention and succeeds then they'll keep at the same thing. Before you realize it you have an addicted teen who can't keep a conversation going longer than 5 minutes. They only talk with abbreviations. Though you might think it isn't too bad and it's possible to live with someone who's constantly on the phone but think about how risky the internet is becoming. Nearly everyone is connected to the internet and all you need is a few minutes or YouTube movies or eBooks for a beginner to know how to hack into accounts. Consider all the negative world citizens your child might come into contact with. The goal isn't to teach your children to not take sweets from strangers, it is about instructing them not to divulge their addresses or any personal information on the internet. They could be at earning children's confidence. Therefore, your child could be at risk on the internet.

It is not my opinion that technology can be a bad thing. It's extremely useful today having the information of the world at the click of your fingertips. I enjoy using social media since I know the best way to utilize it. It allows me to communicate with other people around the world who experience exactly the same issues as I am and have the same beliefs that I have. Social media is truly the most powerful tool that we've had in the past as it allows us to mould our society into the way we would like to see it become. Today, a future in which everyone is treated with equal respect appears more achievable since we are able to work as a whole instead of in a world of divided countries. The technology can be beneficial in the classroom. As as a child I had a back that was in pain from carrying my notebooks, textbooks as well as other school supplies However, now students can access everything with the iPad. This gives them an array of books to pick from, so that they get the most effective education. If technology is employed for the right reasons education, such as in schools and exploring new subjects It is an excellent advantage, however when you use it to allow you five minutes of relaxation and relaxation, it could be damaging to your child's growth as it can increase their feeling of entitlement to grow quickly. The book will also discuss alternatives to "iPad parenting." we'll explore alternative methods to "iPad parenting" that are able to be adjusted depending on your specific situation.

It's not about that children are given technology at an early age that creates an entitlement. Parents using social media can are able to see parents posting photos of their children as well as their experiences with them. The posts are always sugar coated. There is no way to post on how they discipline their children, however they may be extremely disciplined parents (not necessarily that there's something wrong in this). What's wrong is that everything that you see are positive things that lead one to believe that's the way to raise your child. This is exactly the same that models who post swimwear images can affect the appearance of your body since you may wish that you were similar to them. You may feel guilt-ridden about the way you raise your children regardless of whether it isn't financially feasible to take your children to Disneyland or because you don't have the time to take care of the house or look after your children and so, when you take an image, there's always a chaos within the background. Perhaps you were unwell that day and didn't feel like running around the parks with your kids. Don't feel guilty over this. Your child isn't likely to be aware of. Sure, they may beg you to take them to Disneyland But as a child they don't realize how much it costs to simply live. As they grow older, they'll be able to comprehend. They will definitely not care about the mess in your home. Most likely, they won't be bothered, and later, when they are a little older, it is possible to train your children to tidy up little bit. My mother battled cancer while I was a kid but, even though I didn't know what was going on it is always awe-inspiring at the way she raised the kids while being treated. If you're struggling take a breather. You deserve it.

Awakening early to cook the perfect pancakes for your children in order to snap an instant Instagram photo is not realistic for most people. That's okay if use it in moderation. My mother's favourite phrase was "in moderation." But ensure that you do not get into overindulgence because that's where the expectation of entitlement begins. If you give these treats that are Instagram-worthy every day, they'll begin to get used to that. Therefore, think about your kids instead of just your Instagram feed.

Separated or divorced parents are now the norm which is fine. If you and your children are safe and happy is all that matters the fact that they reside together or share a home. Sometimes, however, it can result in an attitude of entitlement. This can start with a broken relationship that isn't resolved or messy. It gets more petty after your child has gone to visit their parents. If you are responding to inquiries with a desire to know what you can do more effective than your ex I'm going to ask you to stop what you're doing now and take a look at your own thoughts. The child you have isn't a nebulous weapon during your divorce fight and you shouldn't make them feel like a weapon. You may be able to buy their a bigger bear right now, but in the future it could be the letting them go at a gathering in defiance of your best judgment, because the divorce decree says that they're allowed to. In order to be clear that a majority times, children and teens will notice this behavior for years ahead of you as they'll use it for their own advantage. It's part of their culture therefore you cannot really fault them for this. One could claim that a parent has no problem with their children not being allowed to leave after the curfew has passed However, it's completely false. Don't fall into this scam. The entitlement process begins when you begin to offer the child everything they desire. You would like to be the most popular, cool or fun parent' however in reality it isn't giving your child anything. If you aren't being the best parent'. You do the exact opposite.

Entitlement Throughout History

It is important to know why entitlement exists so frequently today It is equally important to comprehend why entitlement existed before. This allows us to identify common reasons for entitlement, which will aid us in tackling our modern challenges. That's how we'll become more aware of the notion of entitlement, as well as the personal and social causes of it.

In Europe during the Middle Ages, the Catholic Church ruled due to its wealth and size. In the past, people were required to contribute a 10% of their income to the Church. Also, the church was financially reimbursed for religious ceremonies like weddings, funerals, as well as baptisms. This has become the norm in the modern world. In the end, they controlled around a third of all the terrain across Western Europe, and they were not required to pay tax. Many of the leaders in the church were rightfully entitled and, when they broke the laws and violated the law, the church would defend their rights. In the present, this is similar, sadly since the church's top officials are reluctant to divulge all details they know about specific investigation for them. The reason for this is that, in the Middle Ages, the people belonging to the Catholic religious tradition who started to wander off were branded as atheists and were penalized for their actions. There were those who even sentenced to death. To allow any religious establishment to think that they are entitled to terminate a life due to their lack of belief is absurd. It demonstrates that members in the church were entitled to be protected simply because the church gave the protection they needed, and were richer than the 'commoners.'

A lot of us who consider an earlier time, we usually think of Victorian England with its stunning clothes and homes. The time (around the 1900s-2000s) there was a lot of entitlement. It was generous, though it was only available to the upper class. It was as it currently is a significant disparity in the quality of life from one individual to another. As one person ate each evening a meal of eight courses one sat in the windows, imagining the taste. The most wealthy people of this society did not like those who were poor and considered them to be social scum. They were a shrewd bunch, and often forced their daughters to get married in order to gain more riches. Their privilege was due to being raised in wealthy families, and not having the need to make a sacrifice for wealth and not having to just marry their kids. The poor families were often forced to work for all day in gruelling working conditions only being able to purchase the bare minimum of food needed to provide them with food. A lot of children in poverty died from ailments.

All this happened when the wealthiest people owned large homes that had servants, clean clothes and even a maid. They indulged in food every day, enjoyed vacations occasionally, and indulged their kids with toys. At this point there was a tendency for people of the upper classes would consider that it was unprofessional to offer cash to those who were poor, since being wealthy made people more privileged over those with no money food. That was the most likely period when the concept of the concept of entitlement was especially obvious. Today, entitlement is usually hidden by the person to appear attractive.

From the pop culture, or from history books, everyone is familiar with the reign of Queen Marie Antoinette of France between 1774 and 1793. Marie Antoinette is especially known for her famous quote, "Let them eat cake," as a response to the fact that her people were starving due to the fact that they couldn't afford to buy bread. It is a common mentioned when discussing that the French Revolution because her existence during this period was an influencer in the fight. Her life was lavish. Her clothes were expensive, she consumed a lot of costly meals, held huge parties that lasted for hours, and played huge sums of money. While she was at it the world was who lived outside of her home, starving to their death. The stark contrast between the middle class and the class of the middle classes caused to start the French Revolution. You could go so the extent as to suggest that the greed and entitlement of the wealthy are the reason for their decline. We can see that the wealth of the wealthy plays an important factor in entitlement. Marie Antoinette is probably one of the greatest historical figures who was so privileged.

As you contemplate this, it's why there have been the numerous conflicts and wars all over history. Of the 200 nations in the world, it is the British Empire has invaded every one other 22. And you can you can be certain that they didn't do it in a peaceful manner. The reason for this is that the monarchs as well as the majority of the people of England in the early days decided that they were the most ideal nation and should basically rule the entire world and not care about the freedom of culture, or freedom of speech or even anything else. Hitler also had a right to be entitled. He essentially believed that he was God and decided that a select few were worthy of living if they met his criteria. Naturally, in modern time, we've seen plenty of elected leaders who are entitled. The entitlements of the British throughout history is like the rights of America to us today. America boasts that they excel at anything, but in actual the truth is that they rank quite low in certain regions. The American schools are frequently used as a source of humor in popular culture, however it's clear that these schools are not up to quality of the other countries. One thing is that I cannot imagine how they force children to go to schools in a time full of anxiety, and fear, when they are unable to make them incapable of getting their firearms. Why would you expect anxious students to attend school each day if in some parts of America you have to pass through metal detectors since the people of this country are fond of firearms? In a piece written by Lisa Rose (2018), the United States had 57 times more school shootings as the United Kingdom, Canada, Japan, Germany, and Italy in total. This is an alarming figure. It's possible to say the number of school shootings dropped when Trump was in the White House However, we should not take into account those who did their education at home in the midst of the outbreak. It's impossible to have an attack on a school in the absence of the school.

After we've had an examination of the concept of entitlement both in the past and in the present, we are able to comprehend it in order to rectify this issue that our children exhibit. There is no doubt that the main cause for the difference in entitlement between people of different generations is the amount of wealth. The working-class population is now higher than those from the upper classes. It isn't in the same poverty level as that they had in those times of the French Revolution and the Victorian Era. But, the majority of humanity is in poverty and cannot afford all the basic necessities however it's evident that the vast majority of children's entitlement originates from middle- to upper middle class. Before we can address the behavior and attitude of these children We must ensure that our kids are entitled and it's not something else the reason for their behavior. If you want to know if your child is entitled to it, take a look at the most prominent signs of entitlement among teenagers and children, as well as the signs that are commonly interpreted as entitlement behavior.

Chapter 10: Do You Have An Entitled Teen?

The children who have been labelled believe they deserve all the top of the line and won't accept anything lower. The result will be detrimental on their growth and their later lives. If you've bought this book, you're aware that your child may be probably a bit naughty. You've gotten over the hump--you've acknowledged the fact that your child is entitled and are willing to make changes. If you're still not sure about your child's status there are some basic and difficult signs to consider that you can use for your convenience.

* They don't aid you with daily chores such as cleaning the kitchen or vacuuming regardless of when you request for them to. The chores are essential for children to complete since they will be taught accountability and

develop the abilities they require to be able to leave home.

* They are attempting to transfer the blame to other people when they're caught in a situation that is not their own. My parents believed for a long time that I had eaten the entire box of chocolate at Christmas, but it actually was my brother. It is unlikely that your child will make progress through life if they're continually transferring blame to others; eventually, they'll get arrested.

If you return back from a tiring working day, particularly in the case of a highly stressful job, the people you see aren't affected by the fatigue and stress. Also they don't care about the person you are. They might see your eyes shut, in a state of sleep as you walk in Then they will request that you make their sandwich. While I was a kid I had a mom who worked, and felt stressed as a result. I'd always offer her a hug or massage once she arrived back home, if I was not already in bed. Children need to be aware your feelings, and want to improve your mood like you'd wish to feel happier regarding things. If you fail to impart this knowledge to your child, they could have a child who is very selfish accidentally.

It is possible that your child is entitled when they're completely in a state of being unable to deal with the disappointment. It's normal for kids to shed some tears in the event that they aren't selected to be the winner of the week. However, someone who's entitled may throw an argument about this. Teenagers may be disappointed when their crush begins being with another person, but an entitled teenager will begin making plans for the demise of the crush they're being with.

It is important to encourage them with snacks, money or even toys for basic tasks like cleaning the room in which they live. It's okay to encourage your children to do tasks, but don't be a victim to the trap of thinking, "I'll clean my room when you gift me a reward." ..." my older brother and me used to enjoy cleaning the car of our mother as it was a great family time. Children will be missing the opportunity to experience these experiences when they do only chores to earn reward.

* Many people shun the notion of getting work (if they're old enough for a part-time position). As soon as I turned old enough to get a job I got one. This taught me responsibility as well as interpersonal skills. I could then purchase

things that I wanted to buy, including things to dress up my bedroom. Working also helps teach your child the importance of money and the fact that it's better to save money rather than spend. I think that each teenager must try obtaining an internship when they can. This is a great opportunity that prepares you for the rest of your life. This is an example of my family. My daughter was interested in an iPad at around 10 - or 11-years old. I told her that iPads cost a lot and we didn't have the money to buy one when she was a child. In the months that followed, she asked for one, and we finally agreed. If she were able to pay for half of the price, I'd take the rest. They agreed to save their allowances, and sought out family members for gift cards instead for birthdays or holiday celebrations, explaining her goals and took on extra chores such as yardwork minor renovations, etc. to make and save funds. In the course of a couple of months, she was able to get her reward for all of her effort and hard work. The best thing was she appreciated her reward even more because of all the sacrifices and efforts she put into. The iPad was never any scratches on it, and it was in use until she was unable to upgrade it and she was forced to upgrade.

They always misplace their belongings, and they expect that you do everything to retrieve their items and give the items to them. If I'd left my notebook case in the house I'd have been instructed to borrow a pen from a friend and going, since my parents were both employed a short distance from where I attended school. I was forced to think about all of my belongings, so I didn't have to worry about apology for not having my case for pencils. The child won't be able to explain to the boss that they cannot do their job right now as they're waiting for their friend to pick up their laptop Therefore, teach them how to be responsible to their belongings.

It is a fact that they will always forget what you instruct them to take action. The idea may appear genuine which it is likely to be however, entitled children are likely to not remember what you have told you to do because they are convinced that they don't have to pay attention to the advice of you. This is not a great circumstance if children believe that they don't have to be listening to their parents.

* It could seem like a common sense one However, the kids do not respect the rules that you have set for them, be it you enforce a curfew, or if they are doing

chores. The rules you set are in order to help them learn the value of life, and most importantly all else, to ensure they are in good health. If they don't respect your standards then you're facing a significant security issue, which must never be overlooked.

They will always be wanting to have more, regardless of the amount you offer them. This is commonplace for children, however there's a limit to draw. If you purchase your child a bicycle, but they're unhappy because they want a higher-priced bike, then you've got an issue. When I was young I was a teenager, I was prone to the habit of asking repeatedly whether a reward was meant my treat, even though I was not sure the reason I was getting the reward. The child must be taught that when they accomplish well, they are rewards, however they should not anticipate you to mortgage your home to buy a brand new bike.

In general, once the child turns into a teenager it is also the time to leave temper tantrums, however that isn't the case when it comes to entitled teenagers. It's quite the reverse. I'm not sure if you've ever seen High School Musical, but there's a character from it that's an excellent model of this. Sharpay Evans happens to be a young adult that is frustrated when she does not get her way, will shout and plan her demise on the one that stopped her from gaining her desired outcome. If your teenager has the right to to a certain amount of money, you should be cautious about the cream that they served you, as it could have expired! Don't wish to watch your child who is almost adult get angry because they're permitted to attend an athletic event So, do your part right now to help them get in the right direction.

* They don't have fundamental behavior. It's hard to tell you the importance of manners and how much impact they have on daily activities. Children must know the right way to say thank you and say thank you. The manners of your child will allow them to create a positive impression, although it may seem insignificant right now, it can help in the college interview in the future. If I were a business manager, I'd immediately refuse anyone who didn't possess basic manners. There isn't really any effort to be kind to people around you and practice the proper conduct.

This isn't an exhaustive list or otherwise, this list would be much longer. This is merely a list of aspects that could or may not catch your attention. Of course several other indications you might have observed. The term "entitlement" refers to a child who thinks they are entitled to all the things they want with minimal effort. The result is a host of issues once they reach adulthood and join our modern world, therefore it's best to stop it in the bud as early as possible by being aware of the indicators and improving those behaviors.

It is crucial to remember the fact that there are differences between the genders regarding how the concept of entitlement is displayed. An investigation was conducted by psychologists of Case Western Reserve University and San Diego State University that revealed that sexism was heavily associated with entitlement. The researchers Grubbs as well as Exline (2014) claim that, for males, entitlement has led to a specific view of women as manipulative insecure, and deceitful. Other research has found that this type of attitude was found to boost the risk of female victims being assaulted. Women, for instance, were observed that entitlement causes women to think that men are the ones who should look after them, and they see them and women in general as weak and fragile. The attitude of entitlement makes women less likely to achieve success and progress in any area including working and education. Even though you are unable to discern if this happens to your child at times, it is possible to detect a comment made by a woman which suggests that the entitlement of your child can be seen to your child in the form of sexual sexism. For teenagers, it'll appear more evident to you if they participate with sexism or misogynistic beliefs.

There are times when you can be able to recognize one or two indicators that are listed in the entitlement indicators in children. You might consider, "No, it can't really be the case. This has only occurred a handful of instances." Although entitlement behavior may occur as only a single incident, which is quickly corrected and is never observed repeatedly, if it occurs repeatedly then it's best to begin implementing strategies to ensure that the behavior is not allowed to persist.

You need not fret; you're not the most unpopular parent around. There could be a myriad of causes for your child to become bored and uninterested. In the next section we'll go over the things you could have done to encourage the behavior. Important to remember that you're a human being, regardless of how many children you've have, it's not difficult to fall into mistakes. You must be aware of these errors and adjust your actions accordingly in order so that your child is given the best possible future because entitled behaviour won't aid them in the end time.

Conditions That Can Appear to Be Entitlement

It is possible that you are checking off each one of the bullet points on this list and you get a knowing that you are not an entitlement. There are a variety of conditions that are characterized by symptoms that appear to be entitlement, but they aren't actually caused by entitlement beliefs. In this article, I'll highlight some of the more common. It isn't easy to identify some of these problems, so if believe your child may have one of them, seek out professional assistance to help determine what's happening for your child. I'd like to point out that in the event that your child is found to have one or more of the above conditions, it's not an issue of correcting the behaviour, but instead aiding your child in showing support. The conditions don't mean your child has been rude, or that something is wrong in the child. Some people need assistance and that's perfectly normal.

Depression and Anxiety

However, they are widespread in our culture in the present, and often seem to be a sign of entitlement since some manifestations can be related to boredom. Depression sufferers typically lack the motivation to complete even the simplest of things. The depressed teens often lock them in their bedrooms and lie in bed for more than normal teens which may come off to you like a lack of energy. This isn't your child's blame for being in this way, therefore seeking to change this behaviour is not going to aid. The best option is to consult an expert or a therapist who can guide you to the correct direction. If you're not sure if the behavior is a result of anxiety, depression or entitlement, talk with your child and inquire about how they're feeling. The children and teenagers who are depressed are likely to talk about emptiness, hopelessness as well as general sadness when asked about what they are feeling. It is important that they share their feelings with your story honestly. Some youngsters may not wish to bother you or think that they are able to deal through it on their own. It's vital that you seek out help for your child when they feel depressed as it could lead to suicidal thoughts or tendencies.

Additional signs of depression that are not related to entitlement include:

* Low energy

* excessively sleeping or even not sleeping in any way

* poor concentration

• losing curiosity in the things they were passionate about

• low self-esteem

Physical aches and pains without cause

* posing questions regarding death or being intrigued by death

If your teen or child has any of the symptoms listed above you should to consult with the mental health professionals in order to obtain the support they require.

Nearly everyone experiences anxiety. However, some people are have more anxiety than other. Everyone is anxious, but if anxiety is preventing people from doing something and you are unable to do them, then there's an issue. Teenagers are particularly susceptible to anxiety because it is the time of their lives that is marked by huge changes as well as general awkwardness. In the present, it's especially common in teens because there's a great deal of confusion and changes because of the COVID-19 epidemic. If your teenager is struggling with anxiety, it is possible to believe that they are lazy, and they don't want to do things. It is important to ask your child to justify their reasons they are anxious, since those who suffer from anxiety tend to believe that something negative could happen if they choose to perform the task. Teenagers who feel lazy and entitled will walk out in a fury or stomp their feet, and say "because I don't want to." The people who are anxious tend to fidget, suffer from the sensation of having a heart racing, difficulty sleeping or the tendency to sweat. If your child exhibits such symptoms, it's likely that they suffer from anxiety. get help from a professional in order to learn to manage their anxiety, rather than letting the anxiety take over them and hinder their ability to live the life they desire to lead.

Oppositional Defiant Disorder (ODD)

Perhaps you think your child is rude, entitled and, in general, poorly behaved If they exhibit an ongoing pattern of aggression or irritability, rebellion, or a rage towards the person in charge or others They may be suffering from oppositional defiant disorder, or more simply, ODD. To distinguish ODD from normal bad behaviors, it's essential to document how often and for how long this behaviour is present. In order to be diagnosed with ODD the child should exhibit these behaviors for at least 6 months. If you suspect that your child is suffering from ODD or ODD-related symptoms, it's advised to purchase your own small journal to record each of the behavior patterns you notice on a daily basis in your child and a doctor can diagnose your child more accurately.

ODD could be confused with entitlement since the primary indicators of ODD is a refusal to adhere to the rules, fighting or becoming irritable and angry. The symptoms of ODD are similar to the signs of entitlement, which causes your child to behave this way because they feel entitled convictions are threatened by outside influencers. What is different is the reason why these children are acting in this manner. Unbelief and the belief that a child thinks they are more superior than the rest of us, but there's nothing to blame in the case of ODD. The child will behave this way due to ODD instead of their entitlement belief system. Get medical advice from a professional in the event that you suspect that your child might have ODD.

Highly Sensitive Child

Highly sensitive children can easily be at a loss for words, sounds and even touch. The way they react to stimulus in diverse ways, which range from huge outbursts of anger to mental tumbling, yet their physical appearance remains unaffected. A good example of a hypersensitive child reacting a person passing by them could result in them feeling that someone has hit them with intent. The child could react through a physical punch, becoming angry, or separating their attention from the incident typically in a calm approach. Children who are highly sensitive are highly aware of their peers' emotional reactions, sometimes in the sense that they can't watch a sad movie and not feel that it is happening to their own. The indicators of a sensitive child include:

* perceptiveness

* preferring to play quietly in their own space rather than play together.

* Being shy, quiet or emotionally overtly

* Rapidly reacting to stimulus

* experiencing intense reactions when they feel emotions they experience

* being overwhelmed by crowds or by loud sound

If a child who is extremely sensitive responds in a way that is more extreme than their underreaction It is often mistaken for entitlement. Some children react to events, for instance, the person who is passing them with anger. This may be misinterpreted as anger of people who have a feeling of entitlement. If your child also reacts to sounds that you only hear, as well as to other feelings or specific materials such as certain materials, it might be beneficial seeking advice from an expert.

Post-Traumatic Stress Disorder (PTSD)

It's a tragic event when a young person particularly suffers from the condition of PTSD. This happens because it's result of a traumatizing event as well as the anxiety that comes with it. It's so difficult to think about everything which could have transpired for a child and caused the trauma. It could be any thing, such as a crash in a vehicle or the death of a beloved one or even something more serious. Parents may misinterpret PTSD as a right to entitlement, because they don't know that an event that was traumatic took place. The reason could be that an immediate family member or family member was involved in the incident and did not disclose the event or, if it was someone else, they made the child promise to not divulge the details, or you were not present when the event took place.

The PTSD condition can lead to depression. For teens, it could cause substance abuse as well as violation of laws. Depression can make many people feel hopeless for the future. Therefore, a young person may commit these harmful actions because they believe they don't care about how things go. The trauma of events may make someone feel helpless, lonely and in a state of despair that makes it difficult to carry further. However, the difference situation when it's triggered by an entitlement mindset is the fact that they behave like this because they are convinced they won't be caught or being punished. Teens suffering from PTSD might use substances to ease the suffering as well as the recollection of the incident. For children who are younger fights and anger may be a sign of PTSD. This can also be distinguished from entitlement when you inquire about the reason for this. Children affected by PTSD cannot be capable of identifying an explanation for their anger, as it is triggered randomly because of PTSD while those who suffer from entitled tend to do the act because of someone who resented their entitlement ideology.

The symptoms of PTSD that are not connected to entitlement for children who are under five may be:

Reluctance to let go of the parent or caretaker

* Tense

* speaking but not talking

* sat still for long durations of time

* saturating the mattress

They are displaying behaviors such as chewing their thumbs, sucking their nails, etc.

* appearing older than they actually are

* showing evidence of developing fears that they didn't prior to

When older children aren't teenagers, PTSD may be manifested by:

* areolating their own

* losing interest in the things they once loved

* developing new fears

* grades that are declining

* Feelings of guilt that last forever

• experiencing discomfort and pain without a physical injury to support it

For teens, PTSD symptoms can include:

* flashbacks of the traumatizing incident

* panic attacks

* Substance abuse

* Isolation

• losing enthusiasm for the activities

* Anxiety

* an increase in aggression

* suicidal ideas

* Self-destructive behavior

* participating in dangerous activities

* avoid people, places or things that may bring back memories of the incident

* experiencing sleep disturbances

* retribution wishes

* Guilt

It is vital that you support your child who is having trouble with PTSD with expert help in managing the symptoms and improve.

Attention Deficit Hyperactivity Disorder (ADHD) and Attention Deficit Disorder (ADD)

ADHD is a complex condition that can affect a child's progress in the classroom and their personal relationships. ADHD is often difficult to recognize because it is different among genders. The boys with ADHD typically get diagnosed in the beginning, while for girls, they could become twenties by the time they are diagnosed. The majority of ADHD symptoms are remarkably similar to the symptoms of entitlement. Kids with ADHD often interrupt their peers and struggle to wait their turn. This can be misinterpreted as entitlement. Both entitlement as well as ADHD are able to trigger excessive anger outbursts. Children suffering from ADHD are more likely to throw temper tantrums when faced with demanding situations, like a puzzle that does not have a single piece when entitlement can cause children to behave badly because they desire some thing but can't get the item. The majority of kids with ADHD struggle to concentrate on a single aspect, which is why they be hesitant to engage in tasks that require a long concentration, which could be misinterpreted as lazy that is associated with entitlement in children. The symptom of forgetfulness is of both.

ADD is a kind of ADHD and was reclassified as an inattentive ADHD in the hands of The American Psychiatric Association in the fifth version of the Diagnostic and Statistical Manual of Mental Disorders also known as DSM-5. The condition of Inattentive ADHD is characterized by many of the same characteristics to ADHD and is often misinterpreted as entitlement. A different story that relates to this type of ADHD can be described as follows The following story is about my daughter who has inattentive ADHD (ADD) as well as I observed and continue to see several signs that can be interpreted as entitlement. It was my responsibility to discover the difference and understand that she was not just disobeying me, or flinching in certain instances when I requested her to perform a task. It was it was actually her ADD which caused her to "squirrel"and forget what I wanted from her.

It is crucial for children suffering from ADHD receive an early diagnosis to ensure they receive the support they need to achieve their goals. Signs and symptoms of ADHD that do not relate to entitlement issues are:

* easily distracted, or not paying attention.

* withdrawing from or showing an introverted behaviour

* excessively speaking

* exhibiting increased emotional reactions

* being careless

* spending more time daydreaming than the typical child.

* engaging in risky behaviour

* Having trouble sitting still

* struggling to organize

• having trouble interacting with people

The symptoms of Inattentive ADHD are the ones listed above along with those below:

Losing or misplacing everyday things like keys, or even a cellphones

* prefer activities that have lower concentration

Poor time management

* trouble finishing tasks

It is not an exhaustive checklist. If you think your child has ADHD consult a professional for medical guidance.

Bipolar Disorder

Bipolar disorder is one of the most severe mood disorder. People with bipolar disorder have extreme mood swings, which typically fluctuate between depression and the mania. Both can be considered entitlement-related for various reasons. Therefore, we'll take a the two of them in isolation.

When they are in the depressive phase of bipolar disorder as depression itself, sufferers may become depressed and incapable to accomplish even the most basic of chores. This can be due to the extreme deficiency of motivation, which you could think is lazy. Other signs of bipolar disorder that aren't connected to entitlement include:

* Feeling sad or depressed

* trouble concentrating

* trouble remembering things

* a decline in the interest in previous activities that they had fun with

• having a negative attitude

• loss of appetite

* sleep in excess or no even

* hallucinations

* Suicidal thoughts

Emptiness, or lack of feeling

Manic is perhaps the more apparent sign of bipolar identify. Sometimes, it is mistaken for an entitlement since mania can cause children or teenagers affected by this condition commit risky behaviors like drug or alcohol use or even committing crime. The only exception is when the situation is extremely. There are those who will act impulsively, however, it is usually without causing harm like cutting or dyeing their hair and getting a tattoo from the blue, and so on. The other symptoms of manic moods independent of entitlement:

Feelings of intense joy and happiness

* talking quickly

* huge quantities of energy

* self-esteem

* being easily distracted, or easily angry

* hallucinating

* taking risky or hasty choices that might or might have consequences that are not permanent

* Not sleeping

• experiencing loss of appetite

* uttering words that aren't in the character of the person and that are usually dangerous

If you think your child isn't eligible and instead is experiencing signs of bipolar disorder you must immediately seek medical assistance to assist them discover a solution to living in peace with the symptoms.

It isn't a comprehensive listing of all conditions that could be mistaken for entitlement. There could be numerous things as entitled behaviours. These may not be entitlements however, you may think they are. An excellent example is lazyness. It is a sign of your child's inability to take action, however it is possible that they are physically unable to decide to take the initiative. If you've eliminated these conditions and think your child is struggling with entitlement then read this article to find out what you might be doing to encourage the behavior, and then how you can correct these issues.

www.ingramcontent.com/pod-product-compliance
Lightning Source LLC
Chambersburg PA
CBHW062141020426
42335CB00013B/1291